Disease and Security

Focusing on East Asia, this book sets out a framework for analysing infectious disease threats in security terms. It covers the security significance of naturally occurring disease outbreak events such as SARS and avian influenza, the development and use of biological weapons by state and non-state actors and the security risks associated with laboratory research on pathogenic micro-organisms. The book's main aim is to devise a conceptual framework for securitization that is useful for policy-makers, by using the overlaps and synergies between different infectious disease threats. The book draws heavily on material from public health and scientific literature to illustrate the cross-disciplinary requirements for addressing infectious-disease challenges in security terms. Fast-moving, naturally occurring disease threats are of increasing concern to governments and individuals, and it is therefore important to recognize their close relationship to the security challenges posed by biological weapons and pathogen research. This book will be of much interest to students of international security, public health and Asian politics.

Christian Enemark is Lecturer in International Security at the University of Sydney and Deputy Director of the National Centre for Biosecurity at the Australian National University.

Contemporary security studies

Disease and Security

Natural plagues and biological
weapons in East Asia

Christian Enemark

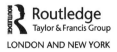

LONDON AND NEW YORK

First published 2007
by Routledge
2 Park Square, Milton Park, Abingdon, Oxon, OX14 4RN

Simultaneously published in the USA and Canada
by Routledge
270 Madison Ave, New York NY 10016

Routledge is an imprint of the Taylor & Francis Group, an informa business

Transferred to Digital Printing 2009

© 2007 Christian Enemark

Typeset in Bembo by Wearset Ltd, Boldon, Tyne and Wear

British Library Cataloguing in Publication Data
A catalogue record for this book is available from the British Library

Library of Congress Cataloging in Publication Data
A catalog record for this book has been requested

ISBN10: 0-415-42234-5 (hbk)
ISBN10: 0-415-56989-3 (pbk)
ISBN10: 0-203-08901-4 (ebk)

ISBN13: 978-0-415-42234-5 (hbk)
ISBN13: 978-0-415-56989-7 (pbk)
ISBN13: 978-0-203-08901-9 (ebk)

Contents

Illustrations

Figure

Tables

Acknowledgements

The completion of this book would not have been possible without the support, encouragement and advice I received from family, friends and colleagues. Thanks first to my loving family – Mary, Stephen, Eve, Damian, Paul, Zita, Phillie, Allan and Damien. From among many marvellous friends, I especially thank Anne Charlesworth, Cameron Crouch, Scott Flower, Vanessa Lai, Rob Law, Catriona McFarlane, Chris Michaelsen, Bernard Mills, Anna Powles, Philippa Reville, Tom Sefton, Duncan Small, Joe Smith, Simon Stone, Brendan Taylor, Helen Thai, Edwina Thompson, Shannon Tow and Moksha Watts. For sharing their thoughts with me on the subject matter of this book, I am grateful to Cheryl Beard, Suba Chandran, Ralf Emmers, Frank Fenner, Rob Floyd, John Gee, Duane Gubler, Adam Kamradt-Scott, Alexander Kelle, Jennelle Kyd, Graeme Laver, Kelley Lee, Colin McInnes, Michael Moodie, Phua Kai Hong, Ian Ramshaw, Jennifer Runyon, Michael Selgelid, Nicholas Sims, Amy Smithson, Joanna Spear, Tan See Seng, Daniel Tarantola, Terry Taylor, Jonathan Tucker, Hugh White and Tony Willis. Of particular value was the detailed advice I received from Des Ball, Richard Brabin-Smith, Malcolm Dando, Alan Dupont, Bob Mathews, Adrian Sleigh and Bill Tow. I am also grateful for the patience and professionalism of Marjorie Francois, Katie Gordon and Andrew Humphrys at Routledge publishing. Lastly, I extend my deepest and eternal thanks to Robert Ayson – an outstanding mentor and constant friend.

Abbreviations

APEC	Asia–Pacific Economic Cooperation
ASEAN	Association of Southeast Asian Nations
BSL	biosafety level
BW	biological weapons
BWC	Biological Weapons Convention
CBMs	confidence-building measures
CIA	Central Intelligence Agency
FAO	Food and Agriculture Organization
IHR	International Health Regulations
NAS	National Academy of Sciences
OIE	Office International des Epizooties (World Organization for Animal Health)
PSI	Proliferation Security Initiative
SARS	severe acute respiratory syndrome
TB	tuberculosis
USAMRIID	United States Army Medical Research Institute for Infectious Diseases
VERTIC	Verification Research, Training and Information Centre
WHO	World Health Organization
WMD	weapons of mass destruction

1 Infectious diseases as a security challenge

At the beginning of the twenty-first century, the threat of infectious disease outbreaks continues to be a serious health concern. However, some aspects of that threat are presently so serious that they warrant treatment in security terms. Accordingly, this book proposes a framework for 'securitizing' a set of infectious disease threats that may arise through natural processes or as a result of human agency, and that have the greatest potential to cause a high degree of damage and disruption in a short space of time. This new, integrated framework is valuable because many security-oriented approaches to infectious disease have hitherto been misguided or inadequate.

To securitize an issue is to lend it a sense of urgency, and to seek some of the overriding political interest and superior financial resources associated with more traditional (military) concepts of security.[1] More than 1,400 species of infectious microbes are known to cause disease in humans, but this book does not propose to securitize them all. Every society tolerates a certain degree of illness such that not all infectious diseases may reasonably be considered a security threat – the mild effects of the common cold, for example, are readily accommodated. Rather, a particular disease may be deemed a security threat when its effects reach the point of imposing an intolerable burden on society. The point at which a disease burden qualifies as intolerable, however, is largely a matter of political judgement. Consequently, the threshold for securitization of a microbial threat may vary from country to country, and from disease to disease. As a general model applicable to any country, this book proposes that the best candidates for securitization are those infectious disease threats that inspire particular human dread, and which therefore generate a level of societal disruption disproportionate to the morbidity and mortality burden they pose.

This approach stands in contrast to the tendency of security scholars and policy-makers hitherto to focus on HIV/AIDS as the highest-profile link between infectious diseases and security. Such attention predates the passage in 2000 of UN Security Council Resolution 1308 which was the first time a health issue had been framed 'officially' as a global security concern. The Resolution expressed concern about the potential adverse effects of HIV/AIDS on UN peacekeeping personnel, but it also stressed more generally that this pandemic, 'if unchecked, may pose a risk to stability and security'.[2] Government policy documents on the topic of HIV/AIDS typically span a range of issues, from how the disease is undermining military capacity to how it is impoverishing millions and destroying social structures vital to internal state security. HIV/AIDS featured prominently, for example, in an influential US National Intelligence Council report on the implications for the United States of global infectious disease threats published in 2000.[3] The following year, however, saw biological attacks in the United States using bacteria that cause anthrax, as well as the publication of a method for genetically engineering a vaccine-resistant poxvirus.[4] The outbreak in 2003 of severe acute respiratory syndrome (SARS) supported further an emerging argument that the security implications of infectious diseases extend beyond HIV/AIDS.

Nevertheless, it would be a mistake to suppose that HIV-oriented models for thinking about disease in security terms can simply be extended to other pathogenic micro-organisms. In a 2005 article, for example, Jeremy Youde sought to 'demonstrate how infectious disease control can be integrated into the three major schools of thought in American international relations theory – neo-realism, neo-liberalism, and constructivism.'[5] In doing so, however, he concentrated on sub-Saharan Africa alone, and on HIV/AIDS alone. Despite this deliberately narrow focus, Youde sought to derive extremely broad lessons: for example, '[b]y incorporating health security concerns *like* AIDS into neo-realism, one can gain a better perspective on how states maintain their survival';[6] and 'AIDS thus impacts many of the concepts that lie at the heart of constructivist theories of international relations, making it invaluable to incorporate disease (and *health security in general*) into international relations' (emphasis added).[7] It is a reality of medical science, however, that there is no disease 'like' AIDS. For reasons such as its long incubation period and modes of transmission, and in the absence of a cure, the virus that causes AIDS is one of a kind. In terms of required medical and public health responses, security-oriented approaches to the AIDS threat cannot simply be transposed onto other infectious diseases, much less 'health security in general'.

The sheer burden of HIV/AIDS, measured in terms of morbidity, mortality and its longer-term social effects, could form the basis for a securitization framework built along different lines. However, this book does not seek to address the security implications of infectious diseases by following a road that is already well-trodden.[8] Rather, drawing primarily on data from East Asia,[9] this book sets out to demonstrate the value of a securitization framework that is limited to three categories of infectious disease challenges presently facing the region:

1   fast-moving outbreaks of natural origin;
2   biological weapons (BW); and
3   the risks associated with research on pathogenic micro-organisms.

Conceptually, and for response purposes, there are extensive synergies and overlaps between each category. The rationale for selecting East Asia as the geographic focus for observation and analysis is correspondingly three-fold:

1   the region has been and is likely to remain the cradle of emerging diseases that spread rapidly;
2   it has a history of state and non-state interest in and use of BW; and
3   the amount of pathogen research being conducted in the region is increasing alongside surging interest in biotechnology generally.

The overall task of this book is to synthesize health and security concerns. The proposed framework for securitizing infectious-disease threats is informed by two disciplines whose language and worldviews are often difficult to reconcile. Disciplinary fences have kept 'security' and 'health' segregated from each other largely because they have represented opposing sets of interests, ideologies and institutions.[10] On one side, the subject matter of security studies has traditionally been death, destruction and military establishments. On the other side, health studies have been about preventing and treating illness, improving quality of life and building up healthcare systems. The value of this book lies in its blending of these two distinct bodies of knowledge, the starting point for which is the mutual concern in both public health and security circles with the need to respond effectively to crises. Infectious disease outbreaks, whether arising from natural processes or as a result of human agency, can be simultaneously a health crisis and a security crisis.

As an introduction to considering infectious disease threats in security terms, this opening chapter is divided into three sections. The first examines the traditional security studies approach of perceiving the significance of infectious diseases in two dimensions:

1   the intersection of disease with issues of armed conflict; and
2   biological warfare.

Beyond the realm of purely military concerns, the second section borrows and adapts some concepts from the Copenhagen School of international security studies and proposes a framework according to which particular disease-based threats could be securitized in their own right. The final section canvasses alternative approaches, from public health and 'human security' perspectives, to the problem of infectious diseases. The chapter concludes with an overview of the concepts and subject matter to be explored in the book.

The traditional view: germs, wars and germ warfare

The background to the securitization framework proposed in this book is that infectious diseases are in many ways already a feature of the traditional security studies landscape. In at least two important areas, thinking about disease in security terms is a far from novel idea. First, it has been and likely will remain the case that infectious diseases are highly relevant to military operations. Second, disease-causing micro-organisms are of obvious military concern when they are spread deliberately as a method of warfare.

Military operations

A good introduction to the way in which infectious diseases impact on security is to examine their relevance to military operations throughout history. Broadly speaking, this can be considered in at least four dimensions. First, there is an abundance of evidence to demonstrate the decisive influence of disease upon battle. For example, the historian Livy described an outbreak of plague in the Carthaginian and Roman armies during the siege of Syracuse in 212 BC. The Carthaginians, less accustomed than the Romans to the city's moist climate, suffered greater casualties from the disease and were defeated shortly afterwards.[11] The sixteenth-century demise of the Aztec empire came about mostly because the Spanish *conquistadores* brought smallpox and measles with them to the New World. And, during the First World War, an outbreak of typhus in Serbia in 1915 was so severe that the fighting on both sides stopped for six months.[12]

The second dimension is that infectious diseases can be of great significance to troop deployments. From the mid-thirteenth century in China, smallpox (which was relatively common among the southern Han people) formed a natural barrier to invasion from the north by Manchurians. When conducting military operations in Han territory, Manchu commanders would deploy only those soldiers who had previously been infected by smallpox and who therefore had lifelong immunity.[13] In the course of the Crimean War (1854–1856), the French sent over 309,000 men east. Of these, 200,000 were hospitalized – 50,000 as a result of battle wounds and 150,000 because of diseases such as typhus and cholera.[14] More recently, in April 2003, Canada's health minister suggested that medical staff from the Canadian forces could help to relieve pressure on Toronto hospital staff treating patients with SARS. The military replied that it was already critically short of physicians to look after its troops, and Canada was at the time preparing for a major deployment to Afghanistan. Had the SARS outbreak in Toronto deteriorated to the point where medical personnel from Canadian military units were required to assist, those units would not have been able to deploy overseas.[15]

The potential for troop movements to spread infectious diseases is the third dimension. In the thirteenth century, Mongol invasions helped to spread various epidemics of plague between East Asia and Eastern Europe. The greatest smallpox epidemic in nineteenth-century Europe broke out when troops were demobilized at the end of the Franco-Prussian War in 1871.[16] And, during the Korean War, American troops were exposed to the

Seoul Hantaan virus – the virus subsequently travelled via troop supply ships to the United States, where it is now endemic.[17]

A fourth dimension of the traditional view of disease and security is the way in which conflict and infection can be mutually reinforcing. For example, the former Director-General of the World Health Organization (WHO), Gro Harlem Brundlandt, has warned of dire consequences if an outbreak of Ebola were to occur in a war-torn part of central Africa. In a conflict situation, it would be too dangerous to send in international health experts to assist in containing the disease, and infected people might start fleeing into cities, neighbouring countries and beyond.[18] Christopher Coker has suggested that the Zimbabwean army, in which many officers have AIDS, was deployed in the Democratic Republic of Congo for the purposes of paying the army's health bills. Given that the average African officer is not paid enough to afford Western AIDS medicine, '[p]illaging a neighbouring state is a way of affording drugs'.[19] And, just as AIDS can be an impetus to war, so too can war cause the disease to proliferate. The most obvious example of this is when soldiers who know they are infected wield HIV as a weapon in the form of rape. In a sense, such soldiers are engaging in a crude, small-scale version of deliberate disease or biological warfare.

Biological weapons

The second major area of traditional security studies in which infectious diseases are of direct military concern is BW. These are pathogenic microorganisms (bacteria, viruses, fungi and rickettsia) deliberately disseminated to cause disease and death.[20] The long history of biological warfare includes plague-ridden cadavers being catapulted over city walls during the fourteenth-century siege of Kaffa, British attempts to spread smallpox to American Indians using infected blankets during the eighteenth-century French–Indian War, and Imperial Japan deploying its extensive BW programme against mainland China before and during the Second World War. On the whole, however, biological warfare has produced very few military successes, and many countries that once maintained an offensive BW capability have since renounced it, including Britain, Canada, France, Germany, Japan, South Africa, states of the former Soviet Union, and the United States. Between them, the various state-run programmes undertook extensive research and testing on many of the biological agents that are common candidates for weaponization: anthrax, plague and smallpox. Elsewhere, however, state interest in using disease for military purposes may persist to this day – US suspicions, for example, typically fall on Algeria, Cuba, China, Egypt, India, Iran, Israel, Libya, North Korea, Pakistan, Russia, Sudan, Syria and Taiwan.[21] Moreover, deliberate disease has also attracted the interest of non-state actors. Examples include the 1984 use of salmonella bacteria by US-based members of the Rajneesh cult, the BW programme run by the Japanese cult Aum Shinrikyo in the early 1990s and the October 2001 attacks in the United States by an unknown perpetrator using envelopes laced with bacteria that cause anthrax.

The latter use of BW against non-military targets is the starting point for moving beyond the traditional approach of regarding infectious diseases as relevant to security only when they intersect directly with war and conflict. Although pathogens can be deployed against military forces, the fact that they could also be used against civilians means pathogens themselves, rather than military operations, can be the core security concern. This is essentially what distinguishes this book from established modes of thinking – it frames certain infectious disease threats as security concerns in a way that does not require, but may include, a military dimension.

As illustrated by the discussion in this section on military operations and BW, infectious diseases are already within the contemplation of traditional security studies. However, for the purposes of security analysis, this book proposes that addressing the problem of infectious diseases can and should extend beyond matters military. Accordingly, the next section describes how particular disease threats may be framed as security concerns in their own right. The focus is on those threats that inspire particular human dread, and which therefore generate a level of societal disruption disproportionate to the burden they pose in terms of illness and death.

Securitizing infectious diseases

Before exploring the notion of securitization, it is worth reflecting briefly upon the meaning of 'security' itself. It is a word that attracts special attention but, if overused or abused, could see its ability to do so diminish. Of particular concern is the way 'security' is sometimes used uncritically as if it always referred to a good thing. Much depends, however, on subjective interpretation. From inside the thick walls of a prison, for example, a person could feel a supreme sense of 'bad' security. A more general approach might be to regard security as freedom from or the absence of threats, but this turns on value judgements as to the nature of 'freedom' and what properly constitutes a 'threat'. Accordingly, this book engages the notion of security as a political construct – an instrument for mustering a greater amount of attention and resources to address a particular problem.

The problem at hand is infectious diseases, the study of which has a natural home in the realm of health. So what is the rationale for extending and elevating certain infectious disease threats into the realm of security? At present, no existing body of theory is of direct assistance for the purpose of framing a response to this question. This book is therefore constructed around disease threats, whether arising through natural processes or as a result of human agency, that have observable political significance sufficiently acute as to stimulate security concerns among people and politicians. These threats are then integrated, with response strategies in mind, according to the overlaps and synergies that exist between them. As such, the ideas in this book are shaped primarily by empirical data rather than an attempt to squeeze facts into some abstract theoretical mould. Nevertheless, it is important to acknowledge the origins and dimensions of the general concept of 'securitization'. Accordingly, the following section explores the extent to which the Copenhagen School of international security studies can provide conceptual guidance.

Some guidance from the Copenhagen School

In a survey of the major schools of international relations theory, Colin McInnes demonstrates that there is little theoretical guidance to be had with regard to linking health and security. Neo-realists, for whom security is about military concerns and the balance of power, see health as a security issue only when it affects military considerations. And although neo-liberals contemplate the possibility of absolute gains for states through cooperation on issues such as trade and security, health is rarely addressed specifically in this literature.[22] Ultimately, McInnes settles on the Copenhagen School as providing an analytical framework most useful for understanding the relationship between health and security.[23] For the purposes of this book, however, the Copenhagen School is a loose fit regarding theory, not least because only recently have a few authors begun to apply its security framework to health issues.[24] Nevertheless, this mode of thinking is useful to the extent that it helps break down some of the key issues at stake when elevating a problem to the security agenda.

The Copenhagen School, originally derived from the work of Barry Buzan, Ole Waever and others at the Copenhagen Peace Research Institute, offers a framework for analysing how a specific matter becomes securitized or desecuritized. According to these authors' approach, any issue can be located on a treatment spectrum ranging from:

- *non-politicized* – the state does not deal with the issue and it is not otherwise a matter of public debate; through
- *politicized* – the issue requires government decision and resource allocation or is otherwise the subject of public policy; to
- *securitized* – the issue is presented as an existential threat, requiring emergency measures that go beyond what would normally be politically acceptable.[25]

Securitization is not, however, simply an extension of politicization. Rather, it is more accurate to regard securitization and politicization as opposites. That is, securitization removes an issue from exposure to the normal bargaining process of politics. For this reason, more security is not necessarily better and could, in fact, make matters worse. In order to analyse the dynamics of securitization and desecuritization, it is therefore essential to avoid the assumption that security is a positive value to be maximized. Instead of

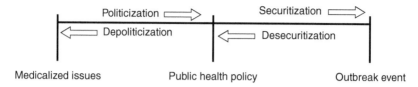

Figure 1.1 Treatment in the health sector.

debating what constitutes a threat, and what ought to be secured, a more appropriate question is: *should* a phenomenon be treated in terms of security? It may often be the case that desecuritizing problems is more desirable than keeping them securitized.[26]

The Copenhagen School model could apply in the health sector, as illustrated by Figure 1.1. Most health issues are medicalized – they are exclusively and non-controversially the business of doctor and patient. Other issues are politicized, which is to say they require government decision and resource allocation or are otherwise the subject of public debate. Health issues that have moved along the treatment spectrum between the points of being medicalized or politicized include tobacco smoking, euthanasia, birth control, abortion and drug addiction. Beyond politicization, particular health issues might be deemed to pose so grave a threat as to warrant securitization.

Returning to the language of the Copenhagen School, for threats to count as security issues they must meet strictly defined criteria that distinguish them from issues that are merely political. Specifically, they have to be 'staged as existential threats to a referent object by a securitizing actor who thereby generates endorsement of emergency measures beyond rules that would otherwise bind'.[27] With regard to infectious diseases, securitizing a particular threat too readily carries the risk of draining attention and resources away from other important areas of health concern. On the other hand, being overly reluctant to securitize might mean a disease threat is allowed to grow to the point where even emergency intervention is futile. This book proposes that the health threats most suitable for securitization are *outbreaks* of infectious diseases – specifically, those that inspire a level of dread disproportionate to their ability to cause illness and death – whether arising as a result of natural processes or human agency. To explore this proposition, the following sections borrow and adapt the Copenhagen School concepts of 'endorsement of emergency measures', 'existential threats' and the 'referent object'.

The dread of infection

The point at which an issue may get legitimately classified as a security problem is a matter of subjective political judgement rather than objective fact. This is because successful securitization is determined not by those seeking to securitize the issue but by the audience from whom they are seeking endorsement of emergency measures.[28] In other words, the critical question is whether securitization is seen as necessary, reasonable and worthwhile by those whose lives would be affected. Paul Slovic and his co-authors, writing in 1980 about risk perceptions, observed that '[society] appears to react more strongly to infrequent large losses of life than to frequent small losses'.[29] They identified 'dread' as a 'higher-order' characteristic of risk which, they argued, correlated closely with a strong societal desire for risk reduction.[30] In its 2002 World Health Report, the WHO referred to these findings and acknowledged: 'The higher the dread factor levels and the higher the perceived unknown risks, the more people want action to reduce these risks, including through stricter government regulation and legislative controls.'[31]

For the purposes of this book, it is important to highlight how the dread associated with some infectious disease threats – individual fear of infection and collective fear of contagion – is a key factor that touches the security nerve of people and politicians. This ancient and visceral dread is what makes citizens of a given country more likely to endorse emergency response measures aimed at protecting them. Heather Schell, writing about narratives in literature, has argued that 'virus discourse imagines the overthrow of the social order. Viruses represent social change – frightening and enormous social change – and our drastic fear of viral epidemics is in part a reactionary response to the possibility of such change.'[32] Writing in 1997, Schell's impression was that 'many people now sincerely believe that the world could end in pestilence, almost as though viruses have now taken the place of nuclear weapons in our apocalyptic imaginations'.[33]

As Jessica Stern has argued, fear is disproportionately evoked by certain characteristics of threats, including involuntary exposure, unfamiliarity and invisibility.[34] With regard to infectious diseases, an infection is always the result of involuntary exposure, and this stands in contrast to the many non-infectious illnesses in which lifestyle choices (for example, tobacco smoking) are a factor. New diseases, or diseases that appear in new places, might produce symptoms unfamiliar to ordinary people, and the fear this generates may be compounded by the inability of medical professionals to provide accurate diagnosis and appropriate treatment. Finally, the threat of infectious diseases is always invisible because disease-causing organisms are microscopic.

When contemplating securitization and the dread of infection, it is necessary to distinguish between what Andrew Price-Smith refers to as 'outbreak events' and 'attrition processes'. For example, outbreaks of bubonic plague (India, 1994) and Ebola (Zaire, 1995) have generated widespread fear and panic, mass out-migrations, military quarantines to contain the exodus of infected people, and considerable economic damage. By contrast, attrition diseases (AIDS, tuberculosis (TB) and malaria) do not generate as much dread as outbreak events, notwithstanding their tendency to result in greater levels of illness and death as well as long-term economic and social erosion.[35] However, because the effects of these diseases are relatively familiar and slow-acting, they do not concentrate the minds of people and politicians as readily as an unfamiliar and sudden outbreak crisis. In addition, the reputation of past pestilences serves to amplify fearful reactions. Between 1896 and 1914, in British-ruled India, bubonic plague (cause of the fourteenth-century Black Death in Europe) killed over eight million people. Over a similar period, TB and malaria claimed the lives of more than twice this number, but it was the plague that generated by far the greatest amount of panic.[36]

In exploring the rationale for giving special attention, in security terms, to actual or potential outbreak events as opposed to attrition processes, it is also worth considering an analogy to war. Why is it, for example, that the military sector is so conspicuous in security studies? And why are military threats traditionally accorded the highest priority among national security concerns? For Buzan, the answer lies in the swiftness with which the use of armed force can inflict major undesired changes: 'Military action can wreck the work of centuries in all other sectors. Difficult accomplishments in politics, art, industry, culture and all human activities can be undone by the use of force.'[37] For Richard Ullman, a threat to security is 'an action or sequence of events that . . . threatens drastically and over a relatively brief span of time to degrade the quality of life for the inhabitants of a state'.[38] In like fashion, an infectious disease outbreak can generate large numbers of human deaths over a relatively brief period of time. Even so, the security significance of such an event lies not simply in the number of people sickened and killed, but rather in the sheer speed at which this human damage occurs. This element of swiftness amplifies the societal dread that attaches to infection, thus generating levels of anxiety and disruption disproportionate to the health burden posed by the disease as it spreads.

Another argument in support of focusing only on outbreak events is that human dread in general tends to garner special political attention, such that the more commonplace dangers in people's lives are less amenable to securitization. Alex Bellamy and Matt McDonald lament the way the threat from 'terrorism' is emphasized over and above the threat from malnutrition. The former, they observe, kills 5,000 people per year whereas 50,000 die from malnutrition every day.[39] This argument nobly assumes one death is worth the same as any other, but it ignores the sensibilities of people and politicians. People are often more concerned with the *manner* in which they might die than they are with calculations of probability. For example, chain-smokers who expressed concern about being killed in a 'terrorist' attack would clearly be giving extra weight to the kind of death they feared more rather than the kind of death to which they are more likely to succumb. With regard to the prospect of infection, people fear some diseases not only because they *can* kill but also because of the *way* in which they kill. Anthrax and Ebola, for example, elicit horrific symptoms such as disfiguring skin eruptions and massive haemorrhaging respectively. Similarly, differing sensibilities can lead to discrimination in the way political leaders respond to security threats. This is starkly illustrated by the UN Security Council's swift response to Al

Qaeda's attacks in the United States on 11 September 2001, in contrast to its prevarication over a series of massacres from April to July 1994 during which 'Rwanda experienced the equivalent of three 11 September 2001 attacks every day for 100 days, all in a country whose population was one thirty-sixth that of the United States'.[40]

Notwithstanding the way securitization may be founded on human dread, it is important to acknowledge that this is a volatile political commodity. Historically, an excess of fear with regard to disease has occasionally led to the overestimation of risks or the design of reactive policies whose costs may have exceeded their benefits. For example, during the Indian experience with bubonic plague from 1896 to 1914, the intrusion of British colonial authorities into the domain of private life was both aggressive and unprecedented. It involved entering homes, meddling with caste and religious practices, and regulating disposal of the dead. The effect of such intervention was often to intensify and quicken the panic occasioned by the disease. This in turn provoked fierce resistance, riots, mob attacks on Europeans and even the assassination of British officials.[41] Admittedly, these late-nineteenth-century efforts to formulate an effective plague policy would have been seriously hindered by general ignorance about the causes and transmission modes of the disease as well as about possible methods of treatment. Today, by contrast, a lot more is known about what causes infectious diseases, and so popular fears may be lessened by the knowledge that effective medical treatment is available. However, the emergence of pathogens hitherto unknown to science can still see people reverting to more primal reactions. For example, despite having caused relatively few human deaths, new diseases like Ebola and variant Creutzfeldt-Jakob disease have tended to generate paranoia, hysteria and xenophobia.[42]

Advances in science notwithstanding, the human dread of infectious diseases can still be compounded by ignorance. The challenge of securitization is therefore to minimize the extent to which irrational fears undermine the practical business of addressing particular infectious diseases. In particular, emergency measures to address outbreak threats must not in themselves jeopardize public safety or curtail human rights to the point that securitization becomes illegitimate. As will be discussed in the next chapter, many public health interventions designed to stop the spread of disease, such as compulsory isolation and quarantine, may appear to infringe civil and political rights recognized in international law. For this reason, and because securitization in general imposes restrictions and expenses on society beyond what would normally be politically acceptable, it is not a move to be advocated lightly. Accordingly, the framework for securitization proposed by this book is strictly limited to three highly-specific and interrelated infectious disease threats.

Disease and security in three dimensions

On the issue of which infectious disease threats warrant securitization, the Copenhagen School approach is to contemplate only 'existential' threats. Thinking about security in terms of survival is what distinguishes Copenhagen School scholars from those who have sought to highlight other imperatives – such as development, humanitarianism and human rights – by using the word 'security'. McInnes, however, departs from the Copenhagen School approach by arguing that requiring an 'existential' threat is setting the bar too high for securitization purposes:

> Issues do not need to pose existential threats for them to be considered security issues. Threats to lifestyle and livelihood have also been widely seen as security issues in that they have the capacity for *extreme* negative effects on individual and social well being, even though they may not directly threaten the *existence* of a social group (emphasis added).[43]

When contemplating infectious diseases, it is more appropriate to follow McInnes in referring to threats as 'extreme' rather than 'existential'. A particular outbreak event (actual or potential) could arguably threaten the functional survival of some states – an example might be pandemic influenza – although there are many others that could readily be perceived in security terms despite not constituting an existential threat. For example, the anthrax envelope attacks of October 2001 in the United States killed only five people, yet few would deny that this incident was a security issue.

The extreme infectious disease threats that underlie the securitization framework for this thesis fall into three categories:

1 biological weapons;
2 fast-moving outbreaks of natural origin; and
3 the risks associated with laboratory research on pathogenic micro-organisms.

As will be demonstrated in the chapters that follow, there are extensive synergies and overlaps between each dimension. For example, there is potential for disastrous laboratory accidents to occur during research into deliberate disease threats, and there can be difficulties in distinguishing biological attacks from natural disease outbreaks. No single dimension of disease-based threats can be considered in isolation from the other two, such that all three must be securitized together.

As discussed in the previous section, BW already occupy a place in the security imagination of politicians and in the academic realm of security studies. However, they tend to be characterized as 'weapons of mass destruction' (WMD) alongside chemical and nuclear weapons. Biological weapons operate on fundamentally different scientific principles and this translates into unique security implications. Most significantly, the effects of a nuclear or chemical attack would be felt immediately. This stands in contrast to the use of biological agents which, because of the time they take to incubate inside human bodies, might not be noticed for days or weeks. The effects of a bio-logical attack have much more in common with those of a sudden natural disease outbreak, and the public health resources needing to be deployed in response would be identical. This book therefore contends that BW should be desecuritized out of the awkward 'WMD' paradigm and resecuritized as constituting one part of a three-dimensional spectrum of disease-based threats.

The issue of BW, already prominent in the thinking of security analysts, is to some extent the hook for bringing naturally occurring disease outbreaks into the security realm. A key consideration is that the consequences of a nat-urally occurring disease outbreak are directly comparable to, and could be as bad as or worse than, a deliberate attack. This was illustrated in a report by two senior officers in the Singapore Armed Forces Medical Corps, Wong Yue Sie and Gregory Chan, on Singapore's experience of the 2003 SARS outbreak. They commented that an 'ideal bio-weapon' is one that is 'easily transmitted and not easily detected, causes severe injury, affects the public psychologically and drains national resources during the response'.[44] Wong and Chan identified SARS as having such characteristics and suggested that an unfamiliar infection would be more difficult to manage compared to a deliberate attack using a known biological agent. This is because, for a new disease like SARS, there are no diagnostic or prophylactic measures available.[45]

Accurate diagnosis and effective treatment of infections, whether deliber-ately or naturally caused, are highly dependent upon laboratory research on the properties of pathogenic micro-organisms. However, this research itself carries security risks. For example, a micro-organism could escape a laboratory because of inadequate safety or it could be stolen by a laboratory worker. Another concern is that pathogen research could lead, unintentionally or by design, to the creation of bacteria and viruses genetically engineered to be more dangerous. The misuse or accidental release from a laboratory of such a 'superbug' could result in a disease outbreak difficult to counter using existing medical countermeasures. Finally, some aspects of state-directed pathogen research may carry international security risks if they are construed by out-siders, rightly or wrongly, as constituting part of an offensive BW programme.

The securitization of three categories of 'extreme' infectious disease threats is an adaptation of the Copenhagen School approach that more readily accommodates the subject matter of this book. As discussed in the previous section, the notion of 'endorsement of emergency measures' is useful in con-sidering how people's dread of infection would make the securitization of these disease threats more acceptable. It remains now to borrow and adapt a third Copenhagen School notion, the 'referent object', to complete the con-ceptual framework presented in this introductory chapter.

Security and the state

The fear and effects of infectious diseases have both an individual and a collective dimension. A pathogenic micro-organism may constitute an 'internal' threat in the sense that it is located within state borders, but also because it inhabits the bodies of a state's human population. It is therefore not obvious whether the individual or the state ought to be designated as the most appropriate 'referent object' of security in the face of such a threat. On this point, it is worth incorporating a public health perspective into a securitization framework – by blending the Copenhagen School approach with a public health emphasis on the health of populations, it is useful to designate the state as a 'rallying point' for security rather than as a referent object. The fact that some pathogenic micro-organisms can kill individual humans is, on its own, insufficient for the purposes of securitization. Death can come to a person from a variety of sources, but to characterize them all as security threats would be analytically unwieldy. Rather, in order for a threat to acquire heightened political significance, something beyond individual harm is required. In the case of actual or potential infectious disease outbreaks, factors such as dread, contagion and the cascading social effects of ill-health quickly elevate the issue from one of myriad individual sufferings to one of broad public concern.

A key problem identified by McInnes is that, whereas foreign and security policy focus on the state as the referent object of security, public health policy focuses on *communities*.[46] Thus it may be that those entities needing to be secured against infectious diseases include individuals and states, as well as communities of individuals that exist inside and across state boundaries. However, dealing with more than one object of security is analytically confusing when contemplating security and organizing effective responses. This book, which places a heavy emphasis on practical response mechanisms directed against deliberate and natural disease threats, therefore rejects the Copenhagen School notion of 'referent objects' in favour of organizational 'rallying points'. And with regard to infectious diseases, it is most useful for combined public health and security purposes to designate the state as the rallying point for action. Although it is true that the invisibility and mobility of pathogenic micro-organisms make them impervious to political boundaries drawn on a map, national borders are nevertheless public health realities. International health agencies like the WHO must operate within a system of sovereign states and, more importantly, they rely heavily upon national governments as the primary providers of healthcare services. At the practical level, once an infectious disease threat has been deemed extreme and therefore suitable for securitization, state-based structures, institutions and resources are of primary importance in resisting that threat.

Designating the state as the security rallying point does not, however, preclude involvement by non-state entities or cooperation between states in defending against actual and potential disease outbreaks. As the December

2004 report of the UN Secretary General's High-Level Panel on Threats, Challenges and Change acknowledged: 'the security of the most affluent State can be held hostage to the ability of the poorest State to contain an emerging disease.'[47] As a consequence, states facing disease-based threats have a strong interest in investing in health programmes and infrastructure beyond their own borders, and in cooperating on international disease surveillance. Today, the increased globalization of human activity allows some diseases to spread faster and further than ever before. Protecting populations against disease outbreaks, whether arising through natural processes or as a result of human agency, is thus necessarily a transnational endeavour. Whereas infectious diseases might in the past have been seen as a security threat simply to the armed forces of competing nations, national leaders need now to recognize the importance of international cooperation against a common microbial enemy.

To place this requirement in historical context, David Fidler offers three perspectives on the pursuit of global health. The first, the *Westphalian perspective*, dominated from the start of international health diplomacy in the mid-nineteenth century (when the nations of Europe began to confront cooperatively the threat of cholera) until the end of the Second World War. This perspective centred on non-intervention in the affairs of sovereign states and framed infectious diseases as exogenous threats to states' interests and power. The second is the *post-Westphalian perspective*, manifested comprehensively for the first time in the 1946 Constitution of the WHO, the Preamble to which includes the statement: 'The health of all peoples is fundamental to the attainment of peace and security and is dependent upon the fullest co-operation of individuals and States.' The central argument behind this perspective is that the fulfilment of the highest attainable standards of health requires that individuals, populations and countries should be seen as interdependent. Regarding the third and newest perspective, *neo-Westphalianism*, Fidler explains:

> Under neo-Westphalianism, manning the barricades of global health is necessary because the germs constitute exogenous threats to a state's national interests, power, and security. . . . Cooperation with other countries and intergovernmental organisations may be required, but cooperation bears no political significance beyond supporting a country's attempts to strengthen its national security, economy, and foreign policy objectives against microbial challenges.[48]

Designating the state as a 'rallying point' for security purposes most closely resembles Fidler's neo-Westphalian perspective on global health. This is not intended, however, to discount or obscure the human dimension of this issue; at the level of practical responses, the ultimate struggle against infectious diseases is played out in the arena of human health and in the bodies of individuals.

Alternative approaches, possible criticisms

Having introduced a framework for the securitization of three overlapping categories of infectious disease threats, the final task of this chapter is to canvass some alternatives to, and possible criticisms of, such an approach. From at least two perspectives, securitizing infectious diseases could be seen as a bad idea. One argument, from a public health perspective, is that securitization might in fact do more harm than good. A second argument, from a security studies perspective, is that infectious diseases are better addressed as a 'human security' challenge.

Securitization: a public health hazard?

In advancing the case for securitization, it is important to acknowledge that infectious disease threats could be securitized in an inappropriate and counterproductive fashion. In Turkmenistan, for example, some infectious diseases were recently elevated to the level of security, and thence consigned to obscurity. In 2004 the country's dictator, Saparmurad Niyazov, declared cholera, AIDS, plague and other diseases to be 'illegal' and forbade any mention of them. The Turkmenistan Anti-Epidemic Emergency Commission stated that there were no cases of dangerous diseases when, in reality, plague was a particular threat in the country at the time. But rather than acknowledge that the disease was a problem, the Turkmen government made its health workers sign a pledge that they would not use the word 'plague'.[49] This case demonstrates that securitization, if not handled properly, can do more harm than good.

With regard to HIV/AIDS, Stefan Elbe warns that, although securitization could strengthen international AIDS initiatives by raising awareness and resources, 'the language of security simultaneously pushes responses to the disease away from civil society toward military and intelligence organizations with the power to override the civil liberties of persons living with HIV/AIDS'.[50] It is less likely, however, that the same objections could be levelled against moves to securitize the narrow range of infectious disease threats discussed in this book. For example, with regard to BW, evidence presented in Chapter 7 indicates that military and intelligence responses are less valuable as vehicles for securitization than are public health responses. And national plans for resisting pandemic influenza are more likely to prioritize vaccination for health workers rather than military personnel.[51]

From a more general perspective, a strong argument against the securitization model proposed in this book would be a humanitarian one; that securitizing particular infectious disease threats would distort public health priorities and result in the neglect of other serious health issues. Recent high-profile events, such as the 2001 anthrax attacks in the United States and the 2003 SARS outbreak, have energized the interest of many countries in infectious disease surveillance, improved diagnostics, and the development of new vaccines and antibiotics to defeat pathogenic micro-organisms. Arguably, this could result in the more commonly occurring problems of human health remaining relatively under-funded. In particular, some public health analysts have complained that resource allocation is being driven by fear rather than a concern to address the diseases that cause the greatest mortality.

McInnes and Lee, for example, object to the recent increased attention to infectious diseases as a 'new security threat' which has mostly focused on selected diseases like SARS, Ebola and monkeypox because they have the potential to move from the developing to the developed world: 'by constructing the links between infectious disease and security in this manner, the global health agenda risks becoming inappropriately skewed in favour of the interests of certain populations over others.'[52] The use of the word 'inappropriately' is an implication that it is *unjust* to distribute resources to such diseases when more common infections such as diarrhoeal disease cause many more deaths. A similar consideration is that infectious disease threats in general, far less those addressed in this book, do not exact as heavy a human toll as do diseases like diabetes, cancer and heart disease, which account for more than 50 per cent of deaths worldwide.[53]

However, it is highly unlikely that a decision to securitize a health problem would be based on simple assessments of the morbidity and mortality burden it poses. In the case of chronic non-infectious diseases, these tend not to garner as much political attention and financial resources as particular infectious disease threats, even in the realm of public health. For three reasons, such diseases are not in themselves as amenable to securitization. First, there is a belief by governments and aid donors that chronic diseases are 'afflictions of affluent populations who have led a life of sloth'.[54] Many chronic illnesses can be attributed to personal choices (tobacco use, poor diet and physical inactivity), whereas no one chooses to be infected by a pathogenic micro-organism. Second, particular features of infectious disease outbreaks – such as disease communicability and the swift descent of illness on the body – generate a greater sense of public urgency. By contrast, a chronic illness may have been building up for many years before reaching the point of threatening an individual's life. Third, because of human sensibilities, non-infectious diseases tend not to inspire the same level of dread. An individual might conclude, for example, that dying quickly of a heart attack is not so fearful a prospect as succumbing slowly and painfully to an infection characterized by grotesque symptoms. Nevertheless, leaving chronic diseases off the securitization agenda does not mean they are irrelevant. In developing countries especially, chronic diseases have added to, rather than replaced, the infectious disease burden – consequently, the strain on health services and infrastructure is all the greater. For example, in China, non-communicable diseases presently account for an estimated 80 per cent of total deaths.[55]

Ultimately, although there is a strong humanitarian imperative to mitigate the potential and actual loss of life resulting from particular infectious disease threats, humanitarian motivations alone are not sufficient. In appealing to national decision-makers, infectious disease threats need to be portrayed in such a way as to stimulate concerns about national interests – historically, governments have shown greater enthusiasm towards their own security than they have towards altruistic causes. Humanitarian appeals can generate a sense of *public health* urgency by citing the morbidity and mortality burdens of numerous health challenges, but it is the dread factor associated with disease outbreaks that touches the *security* nerve of people and politicians. This divide between humanitarian and security concerns is, for some scholars, a problem in itself. As an alternative to the securitization framework proposed in this book, the 'human security' approach characterizes humanitarianism as a security end in itself and therefore seeks to maximize it at every opportunity.

Health and the human security agenda

Concerns about infectious diseases would arguably find a natural home within 'human security' discourse because this is the conceptual space in which much scholarly exploration of the link between health and security already takes place. Feldbaum and Lee, for example, identify two reasons why public health is readily conceptualized in human security terms:

> First, public health and human security share similar humanitarian values and an interest in the well-being of individuals worldwide. Second, the definition of human security includes promoting and protecting health status. There is thus normative and conceptual overlap between the two areas.[56]

At a practical level, however, and in contrast to a framework for securitization, human security offers little guidance on questions such as what threats to prioritize, how and where to allocate resources, and which response measures would be most effective. This problem is largely attributable to the way the human security approach emphasizes the individual over the state as the referent object of security. A common criticism of the human security way of thinking is that if everything that causes a decline in human well-being is labelled a security threat, the term becomes so expansive as to lose any analytical usefulness. An example of this expansiveness is the way Ramesh Thakur interprets the meaning of human security:

> human security refers to the quality of life of the people of a society or polity. Anything which degrades their quality of life – demographic pressures, diminished access to or stock of resources, and so on – is a security threat. Conversely, anything which can upgrade their quality of life – economic growth, improved access to resources, social and political empowerment, and so on – is an enhancement of human security.[57]

At the other extreme, the Human Security Report, published in 2005 by the University of British Columbia, deliberately adopted a 'narrow' approach to human security (focusing on 'violent threats to individuals') so as to make the Report more useful for policy-makers. However, because it rejected a 'broad' approach that would have included 'hunger, *disease* and natural disasters' (emphasis added), the Report offered no conceptual assistance in explaining the security implications of infectious diseases beyond the potential relationship between violent conflict and HIV/AIDS.[58]

The original meaning of human security may be found in the 1994 Human Development Report, published by the United Nations Development Program. This document identified seven dimensions of human security:

1   economic security (assured basic income);
2   food security (physical and economic access to food);
3   health security (relative freedom from disease and infection);
4   environmental security (access to sanitary water supply, clean air and a non-degraded land system);
5   personal security (security from physical violence and threats);
6   community security (security of cultural identity); and
7   political security (protection of human rights and freedoms).[59]

The 'mission' of human security has been presented variously as a means of reducing the cost to human life of violent conflict, as a strategy to encourage governments to address basic human needs, and as a framework for providing social safety nets to impoverished and marginalized people.[60] From a moral perspective, the sentiments driving the human security agenda are unassailable, and the altruism inherent in this discourse is a refreshing shift away from the obsession with self-interest that has characterized traditional security studies.

Human security scholars are good at describing tragedy and lamenting inaction, but not so accomplished at proposing specific policies. A major reason for this is that there is no consensus on what human security is supposed to achieve. For as long as this school of thought is about a multiplicity of lofty aspirations rather than practical solutions, it will ever remain the business of scholars instead of decision-makers. If the human security agenda is too disparate to concentrate the minds of politicians, addressing infectious diseases via this agenda risks having them lost in its dizzying vastness. By contrast, the process of securitization demands unequivocally that a problem be prioritized as a security issue (not as a humanitarian one) and thus compels the implementation of response measures.

Nevertheless, for the specific purpose of addressing infectious disease threats, the human security framework may be more trouble than it is worth. Although the comprehensiveness of human security affords this school of thought great rhetorical appeal, it is unclear how it can guide the practical business of decision-making. Why, for example, should infectious diseases receive more attention than malnutrition or pollution? Such problems affect health security, food security and environmental security. But, without a framework for deciding which is more important, each problem would have to be pursued simultaneously and with equal vigour. And even if decision-makers could be persuaded to concentrate on health security, the problems of priorities and resource allocation within this sphere would remain.

Conclusion and overview

Examining infectious disease threats through a security lens is not in itself a new idea. For centuries, the relationship between disease and the use of armed force has been recognized by military thinkers, along with the possibility of disease being used deliberately in the form of biological warfare. What distinguishes this book is the proposal that the security significance of infectious diseases extends beyond matters military. The securitization framework introduced in this chapter may be summarized as follows:

*   the dread of infection is an impetus towards treating infectious disease threats in security terms;
*   securitization should be limited to extreme threats in three overlapping dimensions (natural disease outbreaks, biological weapons and the risks of pathogen research); and
*   it is most useful to designate the state as the rallying point for responding to these threats.

   The proposal to securitize particular infectious disease threats is open to criticism on public health grounds, and some security scholars might argue that health-related issues are more appropriately addressed through a human security framework. However, it is not necessary for this book to reject outright the arguments that could be directed against it from these alternative perspectives. Rather, such arguments serve as an important reminder that the securitization of infectious diseases should not ignore the inescapable public health and human dimensions of this issue. Ultimately, the value of securitization is that it promises to attract greater political attention and resources for protecting human health and human lives in the face of specific infectious disease threats.

   At the same time, framing particular infectious diseases in terms of 'security' should not undermine the integrity of that concept. If too many problems are framed as security problems, and if security is always presented as a good thing to be maximized, the risks are that security studies loses its disciplinary coherence and that decision-makers might become desensitized. An example of this is the attempt during the early 1990s to highlight the threat of global climate change where, as Gwyn Prins observed, 'the effect of over-selling to try to win the "securitization" bonus was to discredit the scientific underpinning of the entire [climate change] thesis in the eyes of political sceptics.'[61] An important lesson from this experience is that the use of the term 'security' must never be reduced to a linguistic sleight of hand; a ruse intended to fool politicians into caring about something to which they would not normally give priority. By recognizing the need to preserve the special status of security issues, and taking as its geographical focus the East Asia region, this book limits its analysis to three interrelated categories of infectious disease threats.

Part I: Natural plagues

Part I begins with a case study of the 2003 SARS outbreak (Chapter 2) – how countries in East Asia responded, and the lessons for dealing with future outbreak events. Chapter 3 assesses the threat posed by the H5N1 avian influenza virus, which began its transnational spread among birds in late 2003, and the value of measures undertaken or under consideration to prevent or mitigate a possible pandemic of human influenza. The key concerns in this regard are to reduce opportunities for human infection with H5N1 and to enhance local and global capabilities for timely case detection and response if human-to-human transmission of the virus begins. The final chapter in Part I examines the importance of outbreak response capabilities for dealing with SARS-like events and possible influenza pandemics in the future. Such capabilities include access to healthcare, disease surveillance and health system surge capacity. States are central because they are the principal providers of health services, although an effective response to outbreak threats also requires international action. The security imperative for such action is shared vulnerability to contagious diseases in a highly connected world. Institutions offering architecture for effective cooperation against infectious disease threats include East Asian regional organizations, the WHO and the Biological Weapons Convention. The latter is of special importance because of the overlaps and synergies, from a response perspective, between deliberate and natural disease outbreaks.

Part II: Biological weapons

From a public health perspective, the response to an outbreak of natural origin would be largely identical to that required for one caused deliberately. Historically, it has sometimes been difficult to distinguish between the two, but disease control and patient-care imperatives have had to be addressed regardless. From a security perspective, however, it is important to explore how people's visceral fear of infection is amplified by the notion of a disease-based attack by a fellow human. At the personal and political level, humans react differently to the prospect of deliberate disease; it touches the security nerve of individuals and governments in ways that a naturally occurring outbreak does not. Part II is divided into three chapters built on data from East

Asia, as well as broader BW concepts that are not region-specific. Chapter 5 examines the science and history of deliberate disease, with an emphasis on issues relating to state use of BW. Chapter 6 assesses the threat of biological attacks by non-state perpetrators, focusing on motivation and capability as key factors. Lastly, Chapter 7 evaluates military, intelligence, legal and public health responses to the BW problem. Consistent with the lessons drawn from Part I regarding naturally occurring outbreak events, this chapter concludes that strong public health capabilities are the most promising and worthwhile response to BW threats. Another key response to deliberate disease threats, as well as to threats that are naturally occurring, is laboratory research on pathogenic micro-organisms. However, this response is treated as a special case in Part III because of the extent to which research on pathogens generates its own security challenges.

Part III: Pathogen research

Much of the data presented in Part III comes from the US experience of laboratory research on pathogenic micro-organisms that cause disease, although it has direct relevance for any country where such research is going on. Experiments that explore the properties of pathogens have the potential to reveal or enhance medical and public health solutions to outbreak crises, whether of deliberate or natural origin. However, microbiology laboratories also have the potential themselves to be sources of disease-based security threats. Part III explores the risks of pathogen research in two chapters. Chapter 8 examines the need for biological scientists to be more conscious of the security implications of their work, and Chapter 9 is a case study of the security risks associated with the US biodefence programme, from which governments in East Asia can draw important lessons. At present, no country in East Asia has a security-oriented, regulatory framework for managing the risks of pathogen research comparable to that which exists in the United States. This issue needs to be urgently addressed in the region because the number of facilities that store and work with hazardous micro-organisms is increasing. This increase is occurring in the context of biotechnology assuming greater importance in the region's economy, fears that biological attacks might be perpetrated by state or non-state actors and the heavy burden of endemic and emerging infectious diseases in East Asia.

Why is this book important?

This book proposes a much-needed new framework for addressing infectious disease threats in security terms. There are some naturally occurring diseases which, because of their unfamiliarity and the speed at which they spread, pose so serious a threat that they ought not to be designated simply as health issues. The deep human dread of infection that forms the basis for elevating particular natural disease threats to the security realm also applies to BW.

However, there is a tendency among security scholars to perceive the BW threat in 'WMD' terms alongside chemical and nuclear weapons. Rather, solutions to the problem of BW are more likely to be found by recognizing the strong overlap, for response purposes, between deliberate disease threats and threats of natural origin. The best response to both is to strengthen and employ public health tools, the effectiveness of which is vitally supported by research on pathogenic micro-organisms. There has hitherto been little scholarly exploration of the way in which such research itself carries security risks. And so, by addressing pathogen research alongside the closely related issues of BW and natural disease outbreaks, this book brings to the field of security studies new ideas on subject matter which was once almost exclusively the business of biological scientists.

At the beginning of the twenty-first century, natural, deliberate and research-related infectious disease threats are increasingly serious concerns. To inform urgent debate and decision-making, there needs to be a stronger basis of understanding regarding the nature of these problems, why and how they threaten security, and the connections between them. That is why this book is important.

Part I
Natural plagues

2 Severe acute respiratory syndrome

In early 2003 SARS emerged out of East Asia to become the first global disease outbreak of the twenty-first century. This chapter examines the political and security dimensions of the outbreak, with a focus on:

1   how countries in East Asia responded, individually and collectively; and
2   what lessons may be derived from the SARS experience for dealing with future outbreak events.

The first known cases of SARS occurred in Guangdong Province in southern China in late November 2002. On 11 February 2003, the WHO was alerted to an outbreak in the province of atypical pneumonia which had reportedly infected 305 people and caused five deaths. Later that month, a doctor who was inadvertently carrying the SARS virus travelled from Guangzhou (Guangdong's capital) to Hong Kong where he stayed in a hotel. There, the virus was transmitted to local residents and travellers, who in turn transmitted the disease to others when they returned to Vietnam, Singapore, Canada and Taiwan. Within nine months of the emergence of SARS in southern China, the disease had spread to 30 countries around the world. By 5 July 2003, no human-to-human transmission was taking place and the SARS outbreak was declared over. The cost in human lives within East Asia is set out in Table 2.1.

A high fatality rate is often associated with the emergence of a new infectious disease because it is poorly understood, and initial prevention or treatment strategies are absent or ineffective. This in turn can generate heightened concern among people and governments about the personal risk of infection and the collective risk of contagion. As an illustration, the following section examines national and international responses to SARS that took place in 2003 against a backdrop of great social anxiety.

An outbreak event

The SARS outbreak demonstrated the enormous practical and political difficulties associated with containing an unfamiliar contagious disease. In

Table 2.1 SARS-affected countries

Country	Date of first probable case	Total cases	Deaths	Case fatality ratio (%)
China (mainland)	16 November 2002	5,327	349	7
China (Hong Kong)	15 February 2003	1,755	299	17
Vietnam	23 February 2003	63	5	8
China (Taiwan)	25 February 2003	346	37	11
Philippines	25 February 2003	14	2	14
Singapore	25 February 2003	238	33	14
Thailand	11 March 2003	9	2	22
Malaysia	14 March 2003	5	2	40
Indonesia	6 April 2003	2	0	0
South Korea	25 April 2003	3	0	0
China (Macao)	5 May 2003	1	0	0

Source: WHO, *Summary of Probable SARS Cases with Onset of Illness from 1 November 2002 to 31 July 2003* (WHO Online, 26 September 2003). Online, available at: www.who.int/csr/sars/country/table2003_09_23/en/ (accessed 25 September 2005).

Note
Worldwide total: 8098 cases, including 774 deaths.

China, where the disease originated, and in other affected countries, it quickly became clear that implementing public health interventions at the domestic level alone was inadequate. As a consequence, governments in East Asia and around the world were forced to cooperate against a microbial threat that transcended political borders.

China awakes, the region responds

When people in southern China started succumbing to a mystery illness at the end of 2002, the initial response of the Chinese government was to deny the existence of a problem and to refuse offers of assistance from international health authorities. After 15 March 2003, when the WHO issued its first global warning about the SARS virus, China's government-controlled media was prohibited from reporting on the warning. However, just as a contagious disease is no respecter of national borders, it is also impervious to government cover-ups. Already, news of the illness and its victims was circulating around China and the world via mobile phones, email and the Internet.[1] Not until 2 April 2003 was the WHO allowed to visit Guangdong Province to confirm that the alert it had received, nearly two months before, was consistent with cases of an entirely new disease which was by then appearing in hospitals around the world. Later that month, it was finally established that the causative agent was a coronavirus, similar to that which causes the common cold.[2] This discovery meant diagnosis, treatment and containment of SARS could be improved and accelerated.

In hindsight, China was roundly criticized for not cooperating earlier with the WHO, as this probably allowed SARS to spread further. Once shaken out of its complacency, however, the Chinese government then determined to respond to the disease through a process marked by increased transparency and accountability. At a media conference on 20 April 2003, the Chinese Vice Minister of Health, Gao Qiang, admitted to domestic and international journalists that confirmed cases of SARS in Beijing were nine times higher (339 cases) than the health minister's report of 37 cases five days previously, and that the city also had 405 suspected SARS cases in its hospitals. Within an hour of this announcement, the official *Xinhua* news agency reported the removal from office of Health Minister Zhang Wenkang and Beijing Mayor Meng Xuenong. Then, in a speech published on 22 April 2003, Premier Wen Jiabao directed all localities and workplaces to report SARS in a 'timely and accurate' manner – reporting was not to be delayed or concealed, and local and departmental leaders would be held responsible in cases of failure to comply with this directive.[3] Thereafter, China's awakening to SARS propelled the country and its neighbours towards cooperative responses which, for the East Asia region, were extraordinary and in many ways unprecedented.

Beyond China, one of the first countries to appreciate the significance of SARS to East Asia as a whole was Thailand. Although it suffered only nine cases and two deaths during the outbreak, Thailand feared it might incur further damage in the form of trade and tourism losses because people associated every country in the region with SARS. Despite Thai Prime Minister Thaksin Shinawatra promoting Thailand as a 'SARS zero-transmission country' in an effort to limit economic damage, the country was dragged down along with its worse-affected neighbours. Not only was SARS itself a region-wide phenomenon, the damaging power of fear meant all East Asian countries had an interest in defeating the outbreak no matter how little the health of their people was in fact affected.[4]

At Thailand's instigation, the member states of the Association of Southeast Asian Nations (ASEAN) assembled to develop regional responses out of recognition that they all had a stake in limiting the economic and political fallout from SARS. A Special Meeting of Health Ministers from the ASEAN countries plus China, Japan and South Korea (ASEAN+3) was held in Kuala Lumpur on 26 April 2003. The meeting agreed that a comprehensive cross-border approach was the only way to contain the virus. Specific measures agreed to included: studying the feasibility of establishing an ASEAN centre of excellence for disease control; exploring the use of the Internet for information-exchange purposes; and strengthening regional capacity for epidemiological surveillance.[5] Three days later, at a meeting in Bangkok, the ASEAN+3 heads of government approved the initiatives drawn up by the region's health ministers.[6] In addition, on 29 April 2003, the leaders of the ASEAN nations and China met and agreed to implement collectively, and in a transparent fashion, stringent measures to control and contain the spread of SARS. Concrete measures included standardized health screening for all travellers in the region, the establishment of an emergency international hotline, quarantining of travellers that showed symptoms of SARS, and information-sharing regarding the identities and whereabouts of those infected with SARS.[7]

Ordinarily, the adoption of effective regional responses to transnational security threats in East Asia is hindered by the so-called 'ASEAN Way'. Most of the ASEAN member states, highly protective of their sovereignty and territoriality, believe strongly in non-interference and consensual decision-making as core principles of state behaviour in the region. However, following the first meetings on SARS at the end of April 2003, the disease compelled countries in the region to defy the ASEAN Way as their representatives embarked on a frenzy of multilateral, substantive decision-making. On 15–16 May 2003, ASEAN+3 airport officials met in Pampanga in the Philippines and agreed to adopt standardized immunization measures and procedures for preventing the spread of SARS via civil aviation. On 2–6 June 2003, another ASEAN+3 meeting in Beijing agreed to establish effective communications channels, facilitate clearing by customs of medicines and equipment used for the prevention and treatment of SARS, and allow ships carrying a suspected SARS victim to stop at the nearest port for emergency medical assistance.[8] And, in the same month, towards the end of the outbreak, the ASEAN+3 health ministers met in Siem Reap in Cambodia to discuss common strategies for combating SARS and preparations to fight similar outbreaks in the future.[9]

Against the backdrop of this extraordinary regional cooperation, one notable exception was Taiwan. The island, which China regards as a renegade province, is functionally removed from mainland rule, although the two entities retain close commercial links – an average of 10,000–20,000 visitors enter Taiwan from China every day.[10] During most of the period when SARS was spreading, Beijing maintained the position that it was the only legitimate Chinese regime in the world, and that its responsibility to protect Chinese people against the disease naturally extended to Taiwan. Accordingly, China insisted on being the conduit for any requests from Taiwan to the WHO for assistance against SARS, the effect of which was the slowing of crucial communications between Taipei and Geneva. Not until 3 May 2003 did Beijing allow WHO experts to investigate in person the conditions of the SARS outbreak in Taiwan.

Desperate times, desperate measures

Extraordinary responses to SARS at the international level were matched domestically in affected countries by the implementation of societal controls beyond what would normally be politically acceptable. Much of the political concern surrounding this disease was due to the fact that it was unfamiliar to medical professionals and ordinary people alike. Diagnosis was made difficult because the initial symptoms of SARS resembled those of ordinary influenza

– body aches, fever, chills, headache and sore throat – before progressing to a dry cough and breathing difficulties. During the early part of the outbreak, case definitions were hampered by limited understanding of the disease's epidemiology and the lack of a confirmatory test, and because the mode of transmission had not at that stage been determined. Nevertheless, the countries of East Asia erred on the side of caution by presuming SARS was highly transmissible and implemented public health measures accordingly. As a consequence of the fact that no specific vaccine or treatment for SARS existed that would have reduced people's susceptibility to the disease, the only interventions that seemed effective were those that minimized human contact. Transmission of SARS was quickly discovered to be containable using basic measures such as isolation of all infected patients and quarantine of close contacts, but government action also extended to the closure of interstate borders and the use of military personnel to assist in enforcing containment orders.

Singapore, one of the countries worst-affected by SARS, implemented a strategy of containment involving:

1   detection, isolation and containment of actual or suspected SARS cases;
2   protection and monitoring of those not infected; and
3   safeguarding of national borders against those who might import SARS.

Isolation practices were probably the most important component of this strategy. These included converting private hospital rooms to isolation rooms, having a designated ambulance service and 'hot wards' for actual and suspected SARS cases, and restricting inter-hospital patient movements (the disease appeared to be primarily hospital-acquired).[11] Importantly, this containment approach was well-supported by political will. The Singapore government issued over one million SARS kits containing thermometers and facemasks to every residence in the country, and people were regularly stopped at office buildings, schools and other public places for temperature checks.[12] In March 2003, Singapore invoked the Infectious Diseases Act, which empowered the government to isolate everyone known to have had contact with anyone who had fallen ill with SARS. And, in late April 2003, Prime Minister Goh Chok Tong threatened electronic tagging or imprisonment as punishment for people who broke isolation orders.

Similarly, in April 2003, Malaysia's health minister described SARS as a 'national security matter' and threatened prison terms of up to two years for air passengers who failed to declare influenza-like symptoms.[13] Hong Kong adapted a tracing system, previously developed for use in criminal investigations, to map electronically the location of all residences of SARS cases.[14] And Taiwan, along with other countries, established infrared screening devices at two international airports to measure the body temperature of inbound and outbound travellers. Passengers with a fever were prohibited from boarding aircraft, and a hospital near each airport was designated to house, diagnose and treat such passengers.[15] In neighbouring mainland China, the legal and policy measures implemented to combat SARS were among the strictest in the region. Anyone who knowingly spread the disease could have faced capital punishment, and those who broke quarantine or evaded compulsory medical examination or treatment, and accidentally passed on the illness, faced up to seven years' imprisonment.[16] In Beijing specifically, travel bans were imposed to keep the city's residents from carrying SARS to rural areas, thousands of confirmed or suspected SARS patients in the city were isolated, and primary and secondary schools were at one stage closed for two weeks. In addition, the State Council closed movie theatres and Internet cafes, and universities were directed to close their campuses to visitors and to prevent students from returning to their homes outside Beijing.[17]

Living under such conditions, citizens in China and other SARS-affected countries in East Asia may have felt under siege, not only by an unfamiliar disease but also by their own governments. On some occasions, this caused the social anxiety resulting from SARS to manifest itself in civil unrest.

Anxiety and strife

SARS was a security threat not because it killed a large number of people (relative to other infectious diseases, it did not), but rather because a large number of people feared it might. In terms of lives lost, the reaction to SARS was, in hindsight, out of proportion to the health threat it posed relative to other diseases – in China alone, over 100,000 people die each year from TB and there are projected to be ten million Chinese with HIV/AIDS by 2010.[18] But it was the fast-spreading, unfamiliar nature of SARS that inspired dread among individuals – here was a mysterious new illness that seemed able to go anywhere and hit anyone. And the social anxiety and strife that accompanied this impression in turn touched the security nerve of governments.

SARS generated a disproportionate level of fear because, first, there was a lack of medical information about the disease – people knew that SARS was contagious and could be fatal, but the *means* of transmission was far from clear, and there was no cure available. Although surgical masks became the symbol of SARS, they were probably of dubious utility in preventing disease transmission – clinical reports suggested that SARS was spread only by close contact requiring the inhalation of infectious droplets.[19] Second, news of SARS infections and deaths dominated media coverage. According to Caballero-Anthony, the juxtaposition of massive publicity about SARS against the medical unknowns boosted feelings of uncertainty and contributed to occasional overreactions: 'Television and print images of people wearing masks – not just in hospitals but also while travelling on buses, trains, and planes or walking in streets, shopping malls, and other public places – triggered a chain reaction of mass panic.'[20]

In many instances, people's collective anxiety about SARS boiled over into social strife. Around April–May 2003, for example, SARS was associated with large-scale civil unrest and damage to property in many regions of

China. Communities set up blockades to deter outsiders from entering for fear that they carried SARS, and on several occasions peasant mobs attacked and burned quarantine centres that local governments had established in their villages.[21] In neighbouring Taiwan, there was fragmentation and distrust between the central and local governments. When Taiwanese health authorities decided to move some SARS patients from the capital Taipei to Hsinchu city and Hsinchu county, the city mayor and county governor led a crowd of locals to block an ambulance carrying SARS patients to the Hsinchu Hospital. Residents of the city of Kaohsiung, who also feared that the disease would be spread to their neighbourhoods, tried to prevent the opening of a SARS hospital.[22] In Hong Kong, community apprehension reached its peak when it was discovered that a large number of residents from the Amoy Gardens high-rise estate had contracted SARS before the end of March 2003. Most people in Hong Kong live in similarly dense housing complexes, and they were concerned that the cause of the Amoy outbreak was not immediately known. News of the mass infection promoted long queues of people buying face masks, disinfectants and vitamin pills, until soon these items were out of stock.[23] In the adjacent Guangdong Province, police officers were stationed outside supermarkets to restrain panic buying of medicine.[24]

Traumatic as the SARS experience was for people in affected countries in East Asia, it nevertheless served to sensitize their governments to the security significance of outbreak events. Having been forced to engage in international cooperation and domestic intervention to an extraordinary extent, governments can derive lessons from this experience as to how they might respond better to similar infectious disease challenges in the future.

Lessons from the SARS experience

The most important lessons from the experience of responding to SARS in 2003 are:

1   that governments seeking to prevent the spread of an infectious disease deemed to be a security threat should be mindful of achieving an appropriate balance between public health and human rights;
2   that healthcare providers, who occupy the front line during an outbreak, must be well prepared and protected; and
3   that timely communication and cooperation, at both domestic and international levels, are essential to defeating a fast-spreading disease.

Public health and human rights

A number of East Asian countries affected by SARS resorted to voluntary and compulsory isolation and quarantine measures as part of the effort to stop the spread of disease. In many instances, these and other measures would appear to have infringed on civil and political rights recognized in international law. For example, isolation and quarantine affect the right to liberty, disease surveillance potentially affects the right to privacy and travel restrictions affect the right of freedom of movement. However, national leaders seeking to determine a just and appropriate level of intervention can look to international human rights law, which has long recognized that governments may curtail or suspend citizens' rights for public health purposes. With regard to a disease outbreak emergency, the Siracusa Principles provide that

> Public health may be invoked as a ground for limiting certain rights in order to allow a state to take measures dealing with a serious threat to the health of the population or individual members of the population. These measures must be specifically aimed at preventing disease or injury or providing care for the sick and injured.[25]

According to Fidler, to be legitimate under international law, any public health measure that infringes civil and political rights must:

1   be prescribed by law;
2   be applied in a non-discriminatory manner;
3   relate to a compelling public interest in the form of a significant infectious disease risk to the public's health; and
4   be necessary to achieve the protection of the public.

Regarding the latter, the measure must be: (a) based on scientific and public health information and principles; (b) proportional in its impact on individual rights to the infectious disease threat posed; and (c) the least restrictive measure possible to achieve protection against the infectious disease risk.[26]

Ultimately, SARS proved not to be highly transmissible. For example, in Taiwan, by the end of the outbreak, 211,945 people (0.92 per cent of the Taiwanese population) who either had contact with a SARS patient or had returned from a SARS-affected area, were quarantined for 10–14 days. Of these, only 133 were later reported as probable or suspected SARS cases.[27] This does not mean, however, that the extraordinary interventions to contain the disease were unreasonable and illegitimate at the time. Fidler has argued that, on the basis that public health experts initially believed SARS was contagious and could be transmitted through the air from person to person, isolation and quarantine measures

1   appeared to relate to a significant infectious disease threat;
2   were based on the best available scientific and public health information; and
3   were proportional in their impact on individual rights to the serious public health threat posed by SARS and its unchecked spread.

Moreover, the lack of effective diagnostic technologies, treatment options for infected persons or vaccines for prevention purposes suggested that isolation and quarantine measures were the least restrictive measures possible at the time to achieve protection against the spread of SARS.[28]

On the basis of Fidler's analysis, the lesson from the SARS experience appears to be that governments facing this disease-based security threat generally managed to strike the right balance between public health and human rights. However, it is cause for concern that, at one stage during the peak of SARS infections in Beijing, both patients and health workers were locked inside hospitals.[29] Although at the time this may have been a just and appropriate disease control measure, such incidents relate to a second major lesson from the SARS experience – namely, the critical importance of a strong healthcare 'front line' where the health of medical professionals themselves is well protected.

The healthcare front line

Beyond attempting to prevent human-to-human transmission of disease in the first place, the fight against SARS in 2003 was primarily played out in the realm of patient care. During the outbreak, at least two critical factors militated against an effective response:

1   a lack of health system preparedness; and
2   the risk of health worker exposure to the SARS virus.

On the issue of preparedness, developing countries in East Asia were highly familiar with infectious disease problems but lacked adequate disease surveillance and infection control procedures. By contrast, developed countries faced the problem of having had little recent experience of communicable diseases. Indeed, one of the most interesting features of the SARS outbreak was how it exposed the health system shortcomings of two relatively wealthy areas well-connected (in terms of air travel) to the Chinese epicentre of the disease – Hong Kong and Singapore.

In Hong Kong, health professionals had come to regard the territory as relatively safe from infectious disease threats – it had last been declared an epidemic port in 1986, as a result of a cholera outbreak. This attitude was reflected in the fact that Hong Kong hospitals were ill-adapted for managing and treating highly contagious diseases, with very few isolated wards and single rooms. Administrative arrangements in the health system also proved problematic. The Hong Kong Department of Health was responsible for the implementation of health policies, including disease surveillance and control, preventive health programmes, public health education, and family and social hygiene services. But all the public hospitals (which handle over 80 per cent of Hong Kong inpatients) were managed by a separate Hospital Authority. Thus there was no central decision-making body during the SARS crisis, and no clear command structure for healthcare institutions.[30]

Singapore, which enjoys one of the highest standards of health in East Asia, had to learn quickly from initial mistakes made at the healthcare front line. On 22 March 2003 the Singapore Ministry of Health designated Tan Tock Seng Hospital (TTSH), where the first cluster of SARS infections happened, as the national SARS hospital. Management of all potential cases of SARS at one hospital was intended to allow the rest of the healthcare system to function normally. Subsequently, TTSH patients were rapidly discharged to clear beds for the admission of suspected SARS patients, and other hospitals had to carry the load from diverted patients. However, many of the transferred patients were incubating the SARS virus which they had acquired through casual contact with SARS patients at TTSH. This led to epidemics in four of the other five major hospitals in Singapore. The lesson from this experience was that all ostensibly non-SARS patients in the same wards as SARS-infected patients were potentially incubating the virus and would therefore need to be isolated rather than removed to another hospital.[31]

More broadly, Singapore and Hong Kong learned the importance of surge capacity to guard against future outbreak contingencies. In the aftermath of SARS, a 40-room isolation ward at Singapore General Hospital was made ready to admit patients with any contagious disease at any time. And this hospital reportedly also has kept some beds empty in case of a crisis – maximum permitted occupancy is 85 per cent.[32] Similarly, as of August 2003, Hong Kong had spent HK$400 million putting 1,280 isolation beds in nine public hospitals, and HK$100 million retraining medical staff.[33] Even in the midst of the SARS crisis, however, Hong Kong proved it could accommodate a surge in patient demand on an ad hoc basis. At the Prince of Wales Hospital, the epicentre of the SARS outbreak in Hong Kong, many normal services had to be suspended. But to cover the health service shortfall, doctors from the private sector volunteered to carry out surgery for free for affected patients.[34]

The second key issue in treating SARS patients was the need to protect health workers against acquiring the disease themselves. In China, before it was established that patients diagnosed with pneumonia were in fact infected with a new, deadly and contagious virus, hospitals placed them in wards and treated them as they did other patients with the usual forms of pneumonia. This led to the infection of other patients and health workers.[35] Transmission of the SARS virus occurred mainly from face-to-face exposure to infected respiratory droplets expelled during coughing or sneezing, or following contact with bodily fluids during medical interventions. Over 300 healthcare workers were infected within a 17-day period in China during April 2003, and a worldwide total of 21 per cent of probable SARS cases involved healthcare workers.[36] At the very time health systems were struggling to meet patient demand with what few resources they had, hospital-acquired infections were thinning the ranks of medical staff properly trained to diagnose and treat patients.

In the face of significant SARS infection risks, real and perceived, many health workers were unwilling to do their jobs. In Taiwan, for example, where more than 90 per cent of SARS infections occurred in hospitals, over 160 health workers quit or refused to work on SARS wards.[37] Such actions were interpreted partly as resulting from a lack of professional ethics, but they also had a deeply demoralizing effect on Taiwanese society as a vote of no-confidence in the health authorities' strategies for fighting SARS. Some medical workers threatened to kill themselves if kept inside quarantined areas, and there were mass resignations of doctors and nurses at some hospitals. Such events were broadcast to the Taiwanese population at large, leading more people to lose faith in the medical profession and to believe the entire situation was out of control.[38] The lesson from this experience is that the vital healthcare function of treating disease might founder if medical professionals refuse to perform their duties. Safeguarding health professionals against illness and death affords the flow-on benefit of maximizing the availability of medical treatment for the general population. Accordingly, to encourage hospital and other medical staff to attend to their duties during a future outbreak, there should be protective equipment and pharmaceutical treatments set aside for their exclusive use.

Related to the importance of a strong healthcare front line, the next section discusses the third major lesson from the SARS experience: that this front line must be well supported, first, through coordination with other sectors of government and, second, through international scientific collaborations.

Communication and cooperation

Melissa Curley and Nicholas Thomas have observed that a successful national response to SARS required three factors:

1 good channels of communication between medical staff and authorities, between the government and the people, and the extension of lines of communication to and through the private sector;
2 the existence of a high-level, cross-department body which meets daily to coordinate information and policies horizontally across government; and
3 the maintenance of public trust and state legitimacy – something assisted by the first two factors.[39]

Two countries in East Asia that responded in this way with particular success were Vietnam and Singapore. Vietnam, despite its physical proximity to the SARS epicentre in southern China, distinguished itself by bringing the disease under control relatively quickly, and the WHO was able to declare the country SARS-free as early as the end of June 2003. Vietnam reacted swiftly to the disease, placing additional troops on its northern border to prevent the unchecked entry of any Chinese showing SARS symptoms. Of greatest importance, however, was its government's application of high-level leadership early on. An inter-ministerial committee capable of coordinating SARS policy responses across different sectors was quickly established, and the Vietnamese health minister made sure she was easily accessible to the WHO response team deployed in Vietnam and to her own departmental officials.[40]

Singapore, a major regional transport hub, is particularly vulnerable to contagious diseases. Of the lessons Singapore learned from its SARS experience, among the most important was that in a tiny country where the virus could easily and quickly penetrate all areas, a whole-of-society approach is vital. Like Vietnam, Singapore set up an inter-ministerial committee to decide policies that cut across government to deal with all aspects of the outbreak. In order to minimize the social anxiety inspired by SARS, it was vital for the Singaporean authorities to be as transparent as possible and to offer explanations of events in a timely fashion. To this end, the government created a special public-service television channel devoted to SARS, in addition to issuing daily press releases and radio health messages. This stood in contrast to the past experiences of other SARS-affected countries, most notably China, where the revelation of new SARS cases by independent investigations only served to fuel public anger and frustration over government cover-ups. On the whole, the domestic reaction to SARS in Singapore was calm, relative to that witnessed in China. Curley and Thomas attribute this to two principal factors:

1   the government's public control of the outbreak 'agenda'; and
2   the close relationship between government and local media, which allowed the flow of information to be directed.

In addition, beyond direct government dissemination of information, Singapore's private sector participated in the outbreak response by testing the health of company employees daily, and individuals took personal responsibility for monitoring SARS-like symptoms using home detection kits.[41]

In SARS-affected countries in East Asia, the essence of successful national responses was internal cooperation and communication. However, hard-won victories over the disease would have been at risk had assistance not been forthcoming from foreign governments and scientists. The cooperative action taken across the region was itself part of a broader effort against SARS conducted at the global level. In one sense, tighter border controls and travel restrictions might have reflected a temporary, SARS-driven suspension of globalization. At the same time, however, efforts to defeat this disease were facilitated by the free and rapid flow of information between scientists and officials around the world. Just as global interconnectedness enabled SARS to spread as widely as it did, this also led to its demise by allowing information exchanges in three vital areas:

1 surveillance data on SARS cases;
2 information on the best clinical practices for treating and managing SARS patients; and
3 basic scientific research about the pathogenic agent that caused SARS.

The WHO, for example, coordinated a virtual network of laboratories which shared information on a real-time basis through daily teleconferences, thus facilitating rapid progress towards establishing the origins of SARS, the development of laboratory diagnostic tests, and the defining of routes of viral transmission. Such information was a vital tool in the hands of public health and healthcare personnel charged with containing, treating and defeating a disease they had never before encountered.

Conclusion

The security significance of SARS lay in the unfamiliar and fast-moving nature of this deadly disease. In East Asia, hospitals were overwhelmed, trade and tourism suffered, and people's visceral dread of contagion often generated high levels of disruption and instability. The response of governments in the region was to treat SARS as a first order issue of national concern; one which attracted extraordinary interventions against an unforeseen and largely mysterious threat.

At the domestic level, some measures taken to interrupt the chain of disease transmission might, in hindsight, seem excessive. However, a key lesson from the SARS experience is that, in circumstances where scientific knowledge and medical treatments are scarce or non-existent, it is prudent initially to err on the side of caution. In doing so, the actions of governments can be guided and legitimized by the body of international law on public health and human rights. Other lessons from the SARS experience include the need for hospital and health system preparedness, the importance of preventing disease among essential health workers, and the value of cooperation and communication across government sectors. Cooperation was also important at the international level. China's initial reluctance to communicate with international health authorities demonstrated starkly that withholding information only compounds the damage from a contagious disease, hinders the task of containing an outbreak and heightens the risk posed to other countries. In the face of a microbial threat that did not respect national borders, governments in East Asia were compelled to engage swiftly in multilateral, cooperative efforts to halt the international spread of SARS.

From a public health perspective, the positive legacy of the SARS outbreak includes new disease surveillance and reporting techniques, expanded mechanisms for collaborative research on pathogenic micro-organisms, new procedures for infection control, and channels for informing and educating the public about health risks. Beyond these benefits, the levels of emergency response required for SARS and the media attention it generated have served to sensitize people and politicians to the risks associated with unfamiliar, fast-moving disease outbreaks. In particular, the experience of SARS was in many ways a 'dress rehearsal' for addressing the more serious security threat currently posed by H5N1 avian influenza – a disease transmissible from birds to humans which has the potential to trigger a pandemic.

3 H5N1 avian influenza

Pandemic pending?

At the time this book was being written, governments in East Asia and around the world were becoming increasingly concerned about a threat to global security of microscopic size – an avian influenza virus called H5N1. From a health perspective, this virus has a devastating effect on poultry and is highly lethal when it infects humans. The key point from a security perspective, however, is that it might forsake its avian hosts and mutate into a form that enables disease transmission between humans. This situation, although unfamiliar, is far from new. Around 10,000 years ago, when humans first shifted from the hunter–gatherer existence to farming with domesticated animals, settled communities came into close contact with the infectious micro-organisms present in their flocks and herds. This co-existence was the origin of such diseases as smallpox, measles, chickenpox, TB, leprosy, the common cold, malaria, bubonic plague and influenza.[1] In a sense, therefore, the emergence of diseases like H5N1 represents not a new threat but rather a return to 'business as usual' between human and microbe. The key difference is that the stakes are higher in the twenty-first century because increased human interconnectedness could facilitate the global spread of disease.

The prospect of pandemic influenza touches the security nerve of people and politicians in ways that set this disease apart from the many others that may be regarded simply as health issues. A pandemic virus would potentially cause illness and death on a large scale, but that alone is not what excites political attention. Diseases other than influenza exact a great human toll – most notably AIDS, TB and malaria – but they do so in a slow-acting and relatively familiar manner. By contrast, the effects of an influenza pandemic would be swift and unfamiliar. This in turn could generate levels of dread and disruption vastly disproportionate to the likelihood that any given individual would become infected and die.

Individuals have a deep-seated, visceral fear of infection associated with the inherent invisibility of a microbial threat and the notion of horrific symptoms leading to an unpleasant death. In addition, societies have a collective fear of contagion informed by dark memories of past pestilences such as smallpox and bubonic plague. In the case of pandemic influenza, this dread of disease would be amplified by the speed with which damage would occur.

Just as nations fear military conflict because so many national achievements could be quickly undone, so too an influenza pandemic would swiftly set back hard-won economic gains and potentially undermine trust in government. And, like the all-consuming effort of prosecuting a war, defeating 'the flu' would become a first-order issue for governments; one which would alter the premise for all other activity.

Influenza pandemics are rare but recurring. Historically, they have always caused high rates of illness and death, with consequent social and economic disruption. The worst pandemic of the twentieth century was the 'Spanish flu' of 1918–1919 which killed around 50 million people worldwide. Subsequent pandemics in 1957 (the 'Asian flu') and 1968 (the 'Hong Kong flu') were much less deadly, causing two million and one million deaths respectively. Public health experts are now warning that the world is long overdue for another influenza pandemic, and the adverse effects of this coming plague would be all the greater because of increased levels of human interconnectedness – whereas past pandemics spread globally via sea lanes, a pandemic today would spread via international air travel. The conservative estimate of the WHO, using epidemiological modelling based on the comparatively mild 1957 pandemic, is that a future influenza pandemic will cause between two million and 7.4 million deaths worldwide.[2] In early 2006, Warwick McKibbin and Alexandra Sidorenko considered four scenarios for an influenza pandemic. They estimated that a mild pandemic would result in 1.4 million deaths and a cost to the global economy of US$330 billion in lost economic output. The worst-case scenario was 142 million dead and a loss to the global economy of US$4.4 trillion.[3]

There are at least three factors affecting how deadly a pandemic would be:

1   the speed at which the influenza virus spreads;
2   the pathogenicity of the virus; and
3   how much medication is available for victims and potential victims.

A pandemic influenza virus would cause moving waves of outbreaks in humans lasting one-to-two months in a given region and complete its global spread in 8–12 months or less. Eventually, the virus would settle down to cause much milder seasonal epidemics, until the next pandemic virus took over.[4] With regard to pathogenicity, the improved transmissibility required to ignite a pandemic would likely be accompanied by a lower degree of virulence as the virus adapted to its host. That is, the virus in pandemic form would probably not generate rates of mortality as high as have been seen in confirmed bird-to-human H5N1 infections (around 58 per cent). In order to thrive in humans, the virus must not kill too many of its victims too quickly. However, that would also mean estimates of influenza deaths represent only a fraction of the number of people who would be hospitalized, and an even smaller proportion of those who would be infected and fall ill.

On the issue of the availability of medication, it is worth noting first that, in contrast to the situation during the 1918–1919 pandemic, modern antibiotics (for those who can get them) reduce the risk of influenza patients dying from secondary bacterial infections. More generally, however, the main reason past pandemics were so disruptive is because they took the world by surprise. The present situation is different. The world has been warned in advance, with the unfolding conditions for a pandemic under close observation for three years. This advance warning has allowed an unprecedented opportunity for national and international preparation to mitigate the effects of a global influenza outbreak by, for example, researching a pandemic vaccine and securing supplies of antiviral drugs. In addition, the outbreak of SARS in 2003 was a pandemic 'dress rehearsal' which sensitized governments around the world to the health and security significance of a fast-moving, unfamiliar disease.

This chapter assesses the threat posed by the H5N1 avian influenza virus, which emerged most recently in late 2003, and the value of measures being undertaken or under consideration to prevent or mitigate a human influenza pandemic. The key concerns behind such efforts are to reduce opportunities for human infection with H5N1 and to enhance capabilities for timely case detection and response if human-to-human transmission begins.

The story so far

The virus known as H5N1 first appeared in Hong Kong chicken farms in 1997. A total of 18 people were infected and six died in the first recorded instance of a purely avian virus causing respiratory illness and death in humans. Although the properties of the virus were not well known at the time, the killing of all poultry in Hong Kong's markets and farms was a precaution that may well have averted a larger human outbreak of the disease. Thereafter, H5N1 was largely forgotten but not gone. In February 2003, a variant of the virus, similar to one that showed up in wild birds in Hong Kong in late 2002, infected two of the city's residents, one of whom died as a result. Then, on 12 December 2003, South Korea's chief veterinary officer sent an emergency report to the World Organization for Animal Health (OIE) in Paris: a large number of chickens on a farm near Seoul had suddenly died of highly pathogenic avian influenza – a disease never before seen in the country. By early January 2004, reports were emerging of a 'mysterious disease' that had killed thousands of chickens in southern Vietnam.[5] H5N1 had returned and was this time here to stay.

In the months that followed, an epidemic of the H5N1 avian influenza virus swept through East Asia, forcing authorities to cull more than 120 million birds. Although the virus appeared to have been beaten by May 2004, new outbreaks were reported in early July 2004 in China, Vietnam and Thailand. Soon afterwards, poultry flocks in Malaysia, Indonesia, Laos and Cambodia were affected. As of late 2006, the virus had been found in birds in 36 countries.[6] As H5N1 has made its bird-borne journey around East Asia and westward beyond the region, the virus has gradually attracted greater public and political attention. Adding to this, H5N1 has acquired greater significance in the light of human infections with this avian virus and the ways in which governments have responded.

Human infections

Current fears of an influenza pandemic have been excited by the fact that the H5N1 virus has repeatedly managed to jump species and successfully infect humans. Every instance of this is a potential opportunity for the avian virus to mutate into a form better adapted to transmission between humans. As of September 2006, 144 out of 247 confirmed human cases of H5N1 infection had resulted in death, and the overwhelming majority of victims lived in East Asia.[7]

The H5N1 virus already meets two of the three criteria required to cause an influenza pandemic – the ability to replicate in humans and the absence of viral antibodies in the human population. The third criterion is that the virus can spread rapidly among people as easily as regular human influenza. To date, disease in humans has been caused by close contact with infected birds. However, some disturbing evidence of human transmission emerged in late September 2004 in a case surrounding an 11-year old Thai girl who became ill three to four days after her last exposure to dying household chickens. The girl's mother came from a distant city to care for her in a hospital, had no recognized exposure to poultry and died from pneumonia after providing 16–18 hours of nursing care. A study published in the *New England Journal of Medicine* concluded that disease in the mother probably resulted from person-to-person transmission of H5N1 during unprotected exposure to the index patient.[8] And, in May 2006, a cluster of six deaths from H5N1 influenza infection within one Indonesian family prompted an urgent WHO investigation to determine whether the virus had mutated. Fortunately, laboratory analysis of virus samples showed that it had not.[9] Notwithstanding these findings, it is important to acknowledge that H5N1 mutation is not certain to occur. At present, the virus attaches to cells in the lower respiratory tract of humans.[10] It is possible that scientists might discover a feature of this particular virus which prevents it from attaching to upper respiratory tract cells and thus transmitting to others through coughing and sneezing.

Beyond its animal and human health dimensions, the story of H5N1 has also been one of politics. The next section explores how, in the face of a fast-moving and unfamiliar disease threat, some governments in East Asia initially stumbled in their response before recalling the lesson of SARS that international cooperation against contagious diseases is vital.

From cover-up to cooperation

The influenza pandemic of 1918–1919 became known as the 'Spanish flu' because Spain, a neutral country during the First World War, did not have the same restrictions on press reporting of disease outbreaks as did countries still at war in late 1918. Countries today can still be sensitive, for economic and political reasons, about the rest of the world knowing about their disease outbreak status, although such information is now much harder to conceal. One of the most important lessons from the experience of SARS in 2003 was the importance of government transparency in fostering cooperation against a common microbial threat. In particular, China's bungled response to SARS demonstrated how the withholding of information only compounds the damage from a contagious disease, hinders the task of containing an outbreak and heightens the risk posed to other countries. However, some countries in East Asia appear not to have heeded these lessons with regard to H5N1, with the impact of the virus possibly exacerbated by government stubbornness and cover-ups.

Indonesian agriculture officials, reportedly pressured by poultry industry representatives, had for a time insisted that the deaths of at least 4.7 million chickens between August and December 2003 were caused by Newcastle disease, which is harmless to humans.[11] In late January 2004 the Indonesian government confirmed that it had been advised two months previously by senior veterinarians that the country had an outbreak of H5N1. However, according to Agriculture Minister Bungaran Saragih, the government took no action (such as warning international health authorities) because other Indonesian scientists disagreed with the veterinarians' reports.[12] In Thailand, deaths in the chicken industry were still being attributed to poultry cholera as late as mid-January 2004, although it soon emerged that the Thai government had known for some time that H5N1 was to blame. In late January 2004, Prime Minister Thaksin Shinawatra denied the government had covered up evidence of H5N1 and said the health ministry had already been working on the crisis before official confirmation of the disease. He offered the explanation: 'Please trust the government. It did not make an announcement in the very beginning because it did not want the public to panic.'[13]

It is possible Indonesia and Thailand deliberately withheld news of the H5N1 outbreak in their poultry industries. In both cases, political factors may have played a part – Indonesian president Megawati Sukarnoputri might have been afraid of upsetting poultry farmers in an election year (2004), and Thaksin might have wanted to protect Thai exports, domestic consumption and tourism. If so, the strategy of first looking after economic interests may have backfired – Thaksin's public plea to 'trust the government' might actually have stimulated public distrust at home and abroad. On 26 January 2004, for example, the European Union (the second-largest importer of Thai poultry) issued a statement lamenting Thailand's 'nontransparency' and saying that 'complete reliance on Thai assurances does not seem the best way to go forward'.[14]

Immediately after publicly confessing the true nature of his country's problem, the Thai prime minister called a summit in Bangkok to enable regional officials and international health experts to plan a coordinated response to the H5N1 crisis. It would become clear, however, that the delay in official acknowledgement of H5N1 in Indonesia and Thailand had probably precluded timely intervention to stop the virus spreading. By mid-February 2004, the UN Food and Agriculture Organization (FAO) had assessed that cooperation among affected countries in East Asia had improved, with governments realising the paramount importance of transparency in fighting the virus – even reclusive North Korea joined a FAO network of East Asian countries established to fight H5N1 cooperatively in the region. China, Indonesia, Thailand and Vietnam set up information and response structures, but the responses of other affected countries in the region, especially the poorer ones, were from the outset hindered by a lack of resources such as qualified veterinary staff, diagnostic tools and transport.

As of late 2006, these resource deficiencies had not been remedied, such that the poorest countries in East Asia remained the most likely 'ground zero' for a pandemic – wherever the means of detecting and responding swiftly to human H5N1 cases are inadequate, the likelihood of successful intervention to prevent a pandemic is reduced. Accordingly, during what is the first identifiable 'pre-pandemic' phase of history, the two most important areas requiring national and international action are:

1   reducing opportunities for human infection with the avian H5N1 virus; and
2   preparing for damage control in the event that the virus mutates into a form transmissible between humans.

Reducing opportunities for human infection

The first line of defence against the threat posed by H5N1 is to reduce opportunities for bird-to-human transmission. This is important because more cases of human infection mean more opportunities for the virus to mutate into a pandemic form. In most countries in East Asia, the danger of human contact with H5N1-infected birds is increased by traditional practices of raising and handling poultry. In wealthier countries, such as Japan and South Korea, the risk of human exposure is lower because poultry are farmed and sold through intensive, well-regulated commercial operations. However, in developing countries in the region, the level of co-existence between humans and birds is much higher. One dimension of this is the common practice of selling a wide variety of live poultry at markets – these 'wet markets' are potential sites for influenza virus transmission between bird species and from birds to humans. Chinese poultry traders, for example, commonly sleep inside their birds' enclosures to ensure none are stolen. Another dimension of co-existence is small-scale animal husbandry – across East Asia, millions of impoverished families raise poultry at home in order to supplement their diets and income.

Wet markets and small-scale poultry-raising are embedded in the cultures of many East Asian countries. Consequently, efforts to reduce opportunities for human H5N1 infection by regulating such practices have significant political and economic implications. Beyond the basic issue of animal health, government intervention in the region's largely unregulated poultry industry affects the livelihoods of millions of farmers, traders and their families. Nevertheless, the political and economic downsides of intervention must be weighed against the risk that continued human exposure to avian influenza may trigger a human influenza pandemic. Thus far, risk reduction strategies have included culling of infected birds and vaccination of those likely to be infected.

Culling and vaccination

The advantage of culling poultry is that it is the best way to prevent virus transmission from one flock to another. If not carried out properly, however, culling carries a risk of human infection with H5N1. For example, in Thailand at the beginning of 2004, workers conducting the slaughter of birds were provided with masks, caps, gloves and boots, but few wore goggles to prevent infected droplets from getting in their eyes.[15] In addition to wearing adequate physical protection, poultry cullers need to be vaccinated against currently circulating human influenza strains to reduce the chances of co-infection with an avian and a human virus – the possible exchange of genes between the two influenza types inside a human 'mixing vessel' might produce a pandemic virus through a process known as antigenic shift. In any case, by August 2004, the recommended strategy for reducing opportunities for human infection had shifted from slaughtering infected poultry to vaccinating and isolating them. This shift reflected the conclusion of the WHO and FAO that H5N1 was by then so deeply entrenched in East Asia that there was no hope of eliminating it.[16]

Vaccination has been controversial since the earliest days of the H5N1 outbreak. This is mainly because, if not carried out carefully, vaccination may fail to eradicate the virus and thus allow it to make a surprise appearance later. In January 2004, the *New Scientist* magazine published claims that a combination of 'official cover-up and questionable farm practices' had allowed the spread of avian influenza to start undetected in China as early as the first half of 2003. After H5N1 killed six people in Hong Kong in 1997, Chinese poultry producers started vaccinating birds with inactivated virus. If that vaccine was not a good match for the virus, the H5N1 strain may have been able to replicate while causing few animals to show signs of disease. Intensive vaccination schemes may thus have allowed the virus to spread widely without being detected.[17] Although this claim has not been verified, it is representative of broader concerns that fake vaccines or vaccines containing the wrong influenza strain, combined with poor monitoring of vaccination campaigns, could accelerate disease transmission among poultry and thus increase the risk to humans. In wealthier parts of East Asia, vaccination poses less of a risk because it can be closely regulated. For example, Hong Kong's poultry industry, which consists of only 150 farms and a handful of families raising backyard chickens, has an animal health infrastructure capable of monitoring comprehensively the use of vaccines.[18] It is doubtful, however, whether poorer countries in the region have the resources necessary to contain H5N1 in this way.

One such country is Vietnam which, in May 2005, announced it would experimentally vaccinate 600,000 poultry in Ho Chi Minh City against H5N1 – it previously had a strict vaccine-free policy.[19] The difficulty with applying this approach to the rest of Vietnamese territory is that the central government has little way of knowing when and where vaccination (or culling) of poultry is required. Factors hindering the Vietnamese government's goal of eradicating H5N1 from the country by 2010 include the fact that most households keep small numbers of birds that are hard to monitor, and that many animals are smuggled into the country from China, Laos and Cambodia, where disease surveillance is less stringent.[20] In rural areas, Vietnamese farmers have little incentive to report livestock diseases to local authorities because of the absence of insurance or other compensation schemes. In addition, the poorly paid local animal health official who investigates a report of a suspicious chicken death may demand a hand-out from the farmer just for paying a visit. And, in any event, that local official does not have a responsibility to report disease outbreaks to the central government.[21] Under circumstances such as these, where national measures are inadequate to the task of addressing a threat of potentially global proportions, there is a strong case for international assistance.

International assistance

Vietnam, which has shouldered the greatest burden of human H5N1 infection within East Asia, lacks the resources to respond effectively on its own to influenza outbreaks in poultry. In January 2004, for example, Vietnamese farmers reportedly sold as food nearly 800,000 chickens that were supposed to have been destroyed. This may be partly explained by the fact that the Vietnamese government had been offering as little as ten cents in the dollar to compensate farmers who destroyed their chickens.[22] A few days after this was reported, FAO Director General Jacques Diouf appealed to the international community to support compensation payments to farmers in all H5N1-affected areas who suffered losses from killing infected birds.[23] It is uncertain, however, how long a compensation system would need to be in place and whether it is a sustainable response to a virus that now appears endemic in East Asia. Towards the end of 2004, evidence began emerging that ducks could carry H5N1 without showing symptoms and thus could play a role in maintaining virus transmission by silently seeding outbreaks in other poultry.[24] As a consequence, it may now be impossible to eliminate H5N1 among chickens if there is an avian reservoir nearby which does not show it is carrying the virus. Although the FAO recommends that chickens be raised separately from other poultry, enforcing this rule is difficult in East Asian countries where free-range ducks and chickens mingle and share water supplies.[25]

Preparation for damage control

If H5N1 is indeed endemic in the region, the strategy of averting a pandemic by reducing opportunities for human exposure to infected birds is less likely to be successful. As such, an important second line of defence is to prepare early for detecting H5N1 cases if and when human-to-human transmission begins, and to mitigate the damaging health and security fallout from a pandemic. Accordingly, this section examines the laboratory-based disease surveillance and research, the acquisition and use of antiviral drugs and influenza vaccines, and preparation to avoid or mitigate panic and civil disorder.

Disease surveillance and research

The WHO Global Influenza Network, established in 1948, consists of four collaborating centres and 112 institutions in 83 countries recognized as WHO national influenza centres. The network compiles information for influenza vaccine formulation based on the analysis of viral isolates collected in participating countries, and it also serves as a mechanism for alerting countries to the emergence of strains with unusual pathogenicity or pandemic potential. For this network to serve its purpose, however, virus samples must be supplied in a timely fashion. With regard to H5N1, factors that have hampered exchanges between countries and researchers include national pride, intellectual property concerns, lack of political will, safety and security considerations, and inadequate infrastructure.[26] In May 2005, *Nature* reported that it had been almost eight months since the WHO last received data on viral isolates from infected poultry in East Asia, and that it had obtained just six samples from human H5N1 patients. Part of the problem was that the FAO was not sharing what samples it had. More broadly, however, many H5N1-affected countries simply do not have the resources to collect, conserve and securely transport samples of the virus.[27]

In late 2005, the H5N1 virus infected turkeys in Turkey. This attracted the attention of European nations because the virus now appeared to be no longer just an East Asian problem. At a Beijing conference in January the following year, the world's major aid donors, led by the United States and the European Union, pledged US$1.9 billion towards preventing an influenza pandemic. About half of this sum was to be spent in Vietnam, Laos, Cambodia, Indonesia and Thailand on strengthening animal and human disease surveillance, altering agrarian practices, compensating and supporting poultry farmers, improving laboratory and health services, and boosting the communication capacity of these countries.[28] Developing countries in East

Asia are the most likely 'ground zero' for a pandemic, so they require local laboratories (or timely access to foreign laboratories) capable of safely isolating and analysing influenza viruses. In May 2005, for example, laboratory facilities in Hanoi (Vietnam) were so limited that it was taking up to a week for the return of blood test results, by which time influenza patients were sometimes already dead.[29] Because acute respiratory illness can have a number of causes, and early recognition of H5N1 cases is confounded by the non-specificity of the initial symptoms, confirmatory diagnosis requires sophisticated laboratory support. Testing for H5N1 antibodies in a human tissue sample is technically difficult, time-consuming and expensive. And because it involves the use of live H5N1 virus, it should be carried out in high-containment laboratories, of which East Asia has few.

Laboratory capacity is important not only for diagnostic and surveillance purposes, but also because it enables microbiological research to assess the epidemiological characteristics of a disease outbreak and to guide the formulation of effective countermeasures. With regard to the H5N1 virus, knowledge of such factors as incubation period, duration of infectivity and the clinical effectiveness of various medical treatments could guide decisions on whether and how to employ costly and socially disruptive interventions such as limiting human interaction, isolation and quarantine of patients and their contacts, and travel restrictions. Such knowledge would also help to determine the best procedures for diagnosis, sampling and hospital triage, as well as the kind of infection-control measures necessary to prevent disease transmission inside hospitals.

Broadly speaking, however, it is already well understood that public health interventions that were successful in containing SARS are not likely to be as effective against influenza. This is largely because the micro-organisms that cause each disease behave differently – influenza is far more contagious than SARS, it has a shorter incubation period and it can be transmitted at a different stage of infection. For example, infrared temperature-screening devices at airports were useful in the SARS outbreak because people carrying the disease developed fever symptoms before becoming infectious to others. Influenza, by contrast, may be transmissible before symptoms appear. For this reason, quarantine and isolation are also likely to be much less effective at containing influenza than was the case with SARS. Rather, a campaign against pandemic influenza would depend primarily on pharmaceutical defences for individuals. In East Asia, this is reflected in the pandemic preparedness plans of Hong Kong, Japan, Singapore and Thailand, as published by the WHO.[30] Two key components common to each plan are the stockpiling of antiviral medication and mass vaccination. As a vaccine matched exactly to a pandemic influenza strain would take several months to develop and manufacture, the first line of pharmaceutical defence is antivirals.

Antivirals

Pending the arrival of a vaccine, the first concern of governments that can afford it has thus far been to acquire stocks of antiviral drugs capable of reducing the severity and duration of influenza illness. One of these drugs, Relenza, is inhaled. The other, Tamiflu, comes in capsule form and is thus more popular. If taken by a person immediately after he or she is exposed to the virus, Tamiflu can also prevent that person from becoming infected and spreading disease to others. Unfortunately, the world's supply of the drug is limited, largely because there is not constant high consumption in order to treat regular influenza. The exception to this is Japan, which presently consumes three-quarters of the Tamiflu prescribed each year.[31] In the long term, wider prescription of antivirals against non-pandemic influenza would allow pharmaceutical companies to increase their routine manufacturing capacity without fear of losing money. For the present, however, demand far outstrips supply.

Manufacturing Tamiflu is a complex process that can take up to 12 months, from assembling the raw materials to sending out the finished product. Roche, the Swiss-based manufacturer of the drug, quadrupled production between 2003 and 2005, but this did not keep pace with surging demand from developed countries seeking to build stockpiles.[32] In March 2006, Roche announced a series of deals with other companies to increase Tamiflu production that would allow, as of 2007, the production of 400 million treatment courses annually.[33] Nevertheless, for most developing countries, bulk purchases of a drug that costs US$8–US$10 per course (two pills per day for five days) are too expensive anyway.[34]

In the event that large quantities of antiviral medication can be made available before a pandemic begins, plans for damage control must consider how, where and to whom the drugs will be distributed. At the outset, any distribution plan must be accompanied by a commitment to use antivirals appropriately in order to maximize and preserve their effectiveness. One concern is that, if doctors were to prescribe Tamiflu on demand well in advance of an outbreak, individuals would probably use their personal stockpiles in a chaotic fashion, rather than optimally for the purposes of pre-exposure prophylaxis, post-exposure prophylaxis or treatment after influenza symptoms had appeared. In addition, much of the drug would likely be wasted on viral illnesses other than influenza.[35] A second issue, related to the first, is that once tens of millions of people start taking Tamiflu, that drug too might become less effective. In early 2005, H5N1 virus with high-level resistance to oseltamivir (Tamiflu) was isolated from two Vietnamese patients, both of whom died despite being treated with the antiviral drug.[36]

Regarding antiviral distribution at the national level, antivirals would need to be set aside for the exclusive use of two key groups:

1   medical professionals who would be required to keep health systems functioning during a pandemic; and

2   other employees whose work is essential to keep society at large func-
     tioning – for example, supermarket workers, truck drivers, police officers
     and emergency services personnel.

Individual governments would have to decide for themselves exactly who
would be deemed 'essential', and priority-setting for the distribution of
limited antivirals would largely come down to ethical judgements.

In addition, there may be an important international dimension to antiviral
distribution planning. A bold alternative to national antiviral stockpiling
would be to use an internationally run stockpile – Roche has already donated
three million treatment courses (30 million capsules) of Tamiflu to the WHO
– to combat a potentially pandemic virus at its source. If the H5N1 virus was
initially not highly efficient at human-to-human transmission and therefore
spread slowly, there might be a window of opportunity to extinguish it. The
results of a simulation study published in *Science* in August 2005 suggested
that a rapid, targeted response with antiviral drugs at the epicentre of an
H5N1 influenza outbreak in Southeast Asia would have a high probability of
containing the disease.[37] However, there are at least two problems with this
idea. First, the simulation scenario was based on some untested assumptions:
for example, that the influenza virus would not be highly infectious, and that
large quantities of drugs could in fact be distributed rapidly to the right
people, even in remote villages. And, second, even if the WHO were to
recommend a strategy of pooling antivirals, wealthy countries might well be
pressured by their own populations into deciding not to surrender this pre-
cious commodity in response to international cries for help. For example, in
the event of human-to-human transmission commencing overseas, the Australian government has stated that it will 'consider requests from the WHO
or other governments for assistance, and respond commensurately with the
nature of the threat, *without weakening Australia's own capacity* for action should
the pandemic spread here' (emphasis added).[38]

Vaccination

It may be a political reality that, in the event of an influenza pandemic,
poorer countries without antivirals would likely not have access to pharmaceutical defences until a vaccine was available. By that point, the advantage
of vaccinating populations against pandemic influenza would be that it is
much less expensive than administering antiviral medication and more
effective at preventing the spread of disease. The downside, however, is that
the vaccine development process could begin only once the influenza virus
had started to spread, and the disease would probably have circulated the
world before large-scale manufacturing could be initiated. From the time a
virus capable of human-to-human transmission was isolated and analysed, it
could be eight months or more into a pandemic before a matching vaccine
was available.[39]

Developing a human H5N1 vaccine is complicated by the fact that, as this avian virus kills chickens, scientists cannot use chicken eggs in the initial manufacturing process as they do for human strains of influenza. Instead, scientists collaborating with the WHO on this project are using a newer technique known as 'reverse genetics'. The technique has already been used to create candidate vaccines against the H5N1 virus, but the pandemic strain that actually emerges could be so different from the vaccine strains already tested that scientists might have to make a new vaccine from scratch. Alternatively, the candidate vaccine might be sufficiently similar to reduce the severity of influenza illness in humans until a precisely matching vaccine could be produced. In the long term, the ideal scientific breakthrough would be the development of vaccines capable of conferring enduring protection against all influenza virus subtypes and thus of reducing death and disease from both seasonal and pandemic strains.

The hurdles to pandemic influenza vaccine development are political and economic as well as technical in nature. The ordinary situation is that seasonal influenza kills up to 1.5 million people around the world each year as the disease moves between the northern and southern hemispheres. Between 250 million and 300 million doses of influenza vaccine are distributed to the most vulnerable citizens in about a dozen developed countries, and this global vaccine market is worth around US$6.5 billion annually, or the equivalent of 2 per cent of the pharmaceutical market generally.[40] Pharmaceutical companies hesitate to invest in this area because of uncertainty over a viable market, and governments do not go where the market fears to tread because the availability of pandemic vaccines is not considered a public good. This is reflected in estimates that, as of the end of 2005, world capacity for manufacturing a pandemic influenza vaccine was 900 million doses, or enough for only 15 per cent of the world's population.[41] There is little that can be done in the short term to remedy this situation except to build extra production capacity as quickly as possible. However, for this to be commercially worthwhile, there needs to be a long-term increase in consumer demand for vaccines against regular influenza from one year to the next. In essence, a healthy influenza vaccine market would be one constantly primed for a pandemic emergency. Meanwhile, with global vaccine production capacity presently so limited, it is conceivable that people in developing countries in East Asia and worldwide might miss out on vaccines as well as antivirals.

Vaccines, antiviral drugs and laboratory-based disease surveillance and research are each important elements of preparation for damage control from the perspective of human health. However, there remains the issue of limiting in advance the damage associated with the human dread that would accompany an influenza pandemic. In order to minimize societal disruption, it is imperative that the risk posed by H5N1 be communicated publicly. In doing so, the challenge for national governments and international health authorities is to avoid crossing the line between providing information and exciting hysteria.

Pre-empting panic

The effects of an influenza pandemic would be measured not simply in terms of illness and death. In addition, the fast-moving and unfamiliar nature of the disease would inspire dread and potentially stimulate panic within national populations. Under such circumstances, the social contract under which citizens rely on governments to protect them during times of crisis would be subjected to severe pressure. The SARS outbreak of 2003 provided a glimpse of this phenomenon when, in parts of China, there were riots caused by rumours of government plans to establish local SARS-patient isolation wards. Such incidents demonstrate the panic caused when populations imagine a disease out of control, and where governments are seemingly unable to secure the safety of their citizens. On the eve of a possible influenza pandemic, the effects of which would eclipse the 2003 SARS outbreak in terms of both scale and duration, consolidating trust in governments is an essential measure for pre-empting panic.

An example of government squandering of public trust followed the death in February 1976 of a US soldier in New Jersey who had been infected with H1N1 influenza – a disease that had not been seen in humans since 1919. On 24 March 1976, President Gerald Ford consulted some of the world's top virologists and afterwards appeared on television recommending that Congress appropriate funds for a 'swine flu' vaccination programme for all Americans. Within ten months, the United States produced 150 million doses of H1N1 vaccine and vaccinated 45 million people.[42] However, the side-effects of the vaccine killed two dozen people and sickened hundreds of others before the vaccination programme was cancelled. And, because the feared epidemic of influenza never struck, this expensive, unnecessary and occasionally dangerous campaign caused widespread distrust in government health initiatives.[43] The present situation is different because the H5N1 virus, which first emerged in 1997, has repeatedly caused human deaths. Nevertheless, the 1976 'swine flu' experience is a warning against overreaction on the part of governments.

For the most part, the foundation for trust in government during a time of crisis is accurate risk communication before the crisis hits, including reassurance that it might not hit soon, or at all. Accordingly, the WHO Global Influenza Preparedness Plan recommends that governments devise and implement national communications strategies for keeping people informed about the threat of influenza and the measures being taken in response. Such strategies for the 'interpandemic period' include, for example:

- establishing formal communications channels with WHO and other partners for the sharing of information on the genetic evolution and geographic progress of an influenza virus with pandemic potential;
- familiarizing news media with national plans, decisions and activities related to pandemic preparedness;

- maintaining a website with relevant information;
- developing feedback mechanisms to identify the level of public knowledge about pandemic influenza and emerging public concerns; and
- addressing rumours proactively and promptly correcting misinformation.[44]

The last point is particularly important because incorrect information, misinformation or inconsistency in the information available to the public can result in overreactions to media coverage and subsequent internal pressure on governments to respond. Politicians are themselves susceptible to succumbing to the human dread factor associated with infectious disease outbreaks. And, as demonstrated by the 1976 'swine flu' affair, an excess of fear can lead to the overestimation of risks or the design of reactive policies whose costs may exceed their benefits.

As of late 2006, the H5N1 avian influenza virus had not mutated into a form capable of human-to-human transmission, although the risk of this was serious enough to warrant high-level political attention. For the first time in history, governments have an opportunity to warn their citizens in advance of a pandemic, whether caused by H5N1 or another influenza virus subtype. Combined with preparations for damage control in the area of human health, this advance warning should be based upon the best and latest available scientific information being communicated candidly to the public. By thus fostering trust in government, this would do much to minimize the panic that historically accompanies a pandemic. Nevertheless, it is useful to prepare for widespread social anxiety, the imaginable effects of which could include a breakdown in civil order.

Imagining a civil order breakdown

According to the WHO, once a pandemic is underway the overarching goal of national governments should be to minimize its impact. Recommended measures include the following:

- monitor and assess the national impact of the pandemic (morbidity, mortality, workplace absenteeism, regions affected, risk groups affected, health worker availability, essential worker availability, healthcare supplies, bed occupancy/availability, admission pressures, use of alternative health facilities and mortuary capacity);
- assess the need for emergency measures – for example, emergency burial procedures, use of legal powers to maintain essential services;
- inform the public about interventions that may be modified or implemented during a pandemic – for example, prioritization of healthcare services and supplies, travel restrictions, and shortages of basic commodities;
- acknowledge public anxiety, grief and distress associated with the pandemic.[45]

Reading between the lines, the WHO appears to be contemplating the possibility of a breakdown in civil order as societies cease to cope with the enormity of a pandemic. Were this to occur, influenza would become the first-order security concern for governments, overriding all other activities.

In October 2005, the Australian health minister said a pandemic would be 'a test of our national character as well as of our organisational ability'.[46] Implicit in this statement are concerns such as: how would society cope if truck drivers were unavailable and food stopped appearing on supermarket shelves? A critical issue as regards social functioning is whether essential services could be maintained if large numbers of people were falling ill and dying, and more broadly if uninfected people simply refused to risk human-to-human contact. With absenteeism a likely concern, there would need to be ways to maintain services such as healthcare, power, water, food, transport and banking. Historical experience suggests the possibility of other alarming and demoralizing shortages – for example, within one month of pandemic influenza appearing in Washington, DC in September 1918, the disease had killed so many people that coffins and grave diggers were in short supply.[47]

Although it is impossible to predict precisely how public responses to a pandemic would manifest themselves in different countries, it is clear that some governments anticipate severe social disruption. In Britain, for example, contingency plans for a pandemic include posting police at doctors' surgeries and health clinics to stop panicking crowds from stealing antiviral medication. Police would also be placed on standby to prevent public disorder in the event that mass transport systems needed to be shut down or large sporting matches and concerts were cancelled.[48] The 2006 Australian Health Management Plan for Pandemic Influenza provides that 'in the absence of a vaccine, and when containment [through targeted delivery of antiviral drugs] is not possible, Australians should receive the best possible health care *within the context of the maintenance of a safe and secure society*' (emphasis added).[49] And, in the United States, a senior public health official has remarked that the military might be summoned to 'maintain civil order' in the event of an influenza pandemic.[50]

The challenge for governments generally, however, would be to respond effectively and in a way that did not exacerbate public fears. Heavy-handed response measures that do not have a clear public health justification may simply increase panic while doing little to contain the spread of disease. It is cause for concern, for example, that US President George W. Bush has indicated that he would consider using troops to 'effect a quarantine' as part of the US response to a pandemic.[51] Quarantine would likely not be as effective against influenza as it was against SARS because the former can be transmitted from an infected person to others before that person starts to show symptoms. And the sight of troops on the streets may serve only to increase social anxiety during a pandemic.

Conclusion

An infectious disease may reasonably be deemed a security threat when its effects reach the point of imposing an intolerable burden on society. In the case of pandemic influenza, the burden of illness and death would be compounded by the speed with which this unfamiliar disease would move, and in the visceral human dread of contagion that would generate societal disruption. The security significance of the H5N1 avian influenza virus lies in the danger that it could soon acquire human hosts on a global scale. It is therefore in the interests of international health authorities and governments around the world to implement measures aimed at preventing and mitigating a pandemic. One of the most important lessons to be drawn from the 2003 SARS experience is that trans-border cooperation against contagious diseases is vital.

The key concerns are to reduce opportunities for human infection with H5N1 and to enhance capabilities for timely case detection and response if human-to-human transmission of the virus begins. Risk-reduction strategies have so far included the culling of infected birds and vaccination of those at risk of infection, although the poorer countries of East Asia are incapable of sustaining such efforts without increased international assistance. In any event, because initial outbreaks of H5N1 were not contained, the virus has likely become endemic to the region and thus may be impossible to eradicate. This has led to a shift in emphasis away from reducing opportunities for human infection and towards preparation for damage control in the face of a looming pandemic. The most important measures for achieving this are laboratory-based disease surveillance and research, the acquisition and use of antiviral drugs and influenza vaccines, and communication between governments and the public regarding the risks posed by avian influenza. Arguably, the best response to the threat of a pandemic is to respond better to regular, non-pandemic influenza by ramping up vaccination rates. However, this would be a long-term solution dependent upon an expansion of world vaccine manufacturing capacity far beyond what presently exists. In the short term, governments might need to consider guarding against outbreak contingencies by generating demand for vaccine production where the market does not.

Finally, it is important to emphasize the international dimension of the influenza challenge. In contrast to the experience of past pandemics, which were all the more damaging because they burst out with no warning, the world today has an unprecedented opportunity to engage in cooperative intervention aimed at delaying the emergence of a pandemic influenza virus or curtailing its spread. The conditions for an influenza pandemic are close to being realized, and the window of opportunity to prepare may not remain open for long. Against a microbial threat that knows no borders, countries that are presently not directly affected by H5N1 avian influenza must treat this problem as if it were their own. Success against the virus, the cradle of which is East Asia, is heavily dependent upon donors within and beyond the region providing assistance to its most vulnerable countries – those with the weakest health infrastructure. This assistance would most usefully take the form of enhancing disease surveillance networks and strengthening national capabilities for patient care. These and other aspects of outbreak response capacity are discussed in the next chapter.

4 Outbreak response
Rallying around the state

In the aftermath of SARS, and in the context of increasing concern about an imminent influenza pandemic, it is worth considering the general capacity of countries to cope with outbreak events. In terms of human health, the fight against infectious diseases ultimately takes place inside individuals' bodies. From a security and public health perspective, however, it is most useful to designate the state rather than the individual as the rallying point for action – states are central because they are the principal providers of health services. Key aspects of outbreak response capacity examined in this chapter include the level of access to healthcare, disease surveillance capabilities and health system surge capacity. In addition, nationally focused response efforts require international cooperation and coordination against microbial threats that transcend political borders, the security imperative for which is shared vulnerability in a highly connected world. For countries in East Asia, existing regional organizations and the WHO provide institutional architecture for effective cooperation against infectious diseases, as does the Biological Weapons Convention.

National health resources

The backdrop to an outbreak event includes the health resources (human, physical and financial) available to the citizens of a given country. Within East Asia, there is much scope to enhance outbreak response capacity by improving national health system capabilities, with some national systems more in need of improvement than others. The numerical data presented in Table 4.1 indicate varying degrees of human resource allocation by countries within the region, and suggest roughly how well each is positioned to respond to ongoing health problems as well as an outbreak emergency. The caveat attached to these figures is that the skill levels of local health workers may vary, particularly between the developed and developing countries that make up the region. In addition, there are important qualitative differences between East Asian countries that temper outbreak response capacity. For example, in Myanmar, one of the poorest countries in the region, epidemics of cholera, plague and dengue are constantly occurring. The main constraints on resisting these diseases have been the low level of health awareness among the population, poor sanitation, overworked medical professionals, poor health facilities and inadequate transport for supervision of epidemic response strategies. Vietnam, which also suffers from some of these problems, nevertheless has a better-organized health system. Reasons for this include the country's strong central government, and past exposure to French, American

Table 4.1 Human resources for health

Country	Population in 2003	Physicians per 100,000 (year)	Nurses per 100,000 (year)
Brunei	358,000	101 2000	267 2000
Cambodia	14,144,000	16 2000	61 2000
China	1,311,709,000	164 2000	104 2002
Indonesia	219,883,000	16 2000	44 2000
Japan	127,654,000	201 2000	821 2000
Laos	5,657,000	59 1996	103 1996
Malaysia	24,425,000	70 2000	135 2000
Myanmar	49,485,000	30 2000	27 2000
North Korea	22,664,000	297 1995	180 1995
Philippines	79,999,000	116 2002	442 2002
Singapore	4,253,000	140 2001	424 2001
South Korea	47,700,000	181 2000	342 2000
Thailand	62,833,000	30 1999	162 1999
Timor-Leste	778,000	No data	No data
Vietnam	81,377,000	53 2001	56 2001

Sources: WHO, *Global Health Atlas* (WHO Online). Online, available at: globalatlas.who.int/globalatlas/dataQuery/default.asp (accessed 5 October 2005), WHO; *World Health Report 2005: Make Every Mother and Child Count*, Geneva: World Health Organization, 2005, pp. 174–181.

and Russian influences that enabled access to Western medicine. At the richer end of the spectrum, Brunei provides free healthcare for all its citizens and, for medical care not available locally, sends patients overseas at government expense. In Singapore, where a large number of high-quality medical services are available, the government actively promotes preventive healthcare programmes and encourages citizens to take a high level of responsibility for their own health.

In wealthier parts of East Asia, a lack of capacity to resist outbreak threats may be attributable not to the scarcity of health resources but rather to the way in which they are managed. At the time SARS hit Hong Kong, for example, 90 per cent of the territory's annual health budget of over HK$30 billion went to the Hospitals Authority, with the Department of Health receiving less than 10 per cent. This had the effect of directing most resources towards patient treatment, with prevention, public health education and public hygiene of secondary importance.[1] Arguably, greater resource allocation aimed at the prevention of disease prior to 2003 might have placed Hong Kong in a stronger position to resist SARS.

Beyond the broad issue of how much is spent on health in general, this section examines three critical factors that affect a national health system's ability to respond to an outbreak event:

1   the extent to which citizens can access healthcare;
2   disease surveillance capabilities; and
3   the capacity of the health system to cope with a sudden surge in demand for medical treatment.

The section concludes with a case study of China's health resources.

Access to care

Early detection of an infectious disease outbreak is dependent upon people first having access to the healthcare system so that their illness can be reported to public health authorities. Those with public or private health insurance are more likely to visit their doctors at the first sign of illness, whereas uninsured people tend to delay seeking treatment. As indicated by Table 4.2, there is considerable diversity in East Asia on health expenditure, in terms of the level of government health spending and the extent to which a patient is liable for the cost of his or her medical treatment.

An examination of particular countries provides greater insight into differing approaches to health spending across the region. For example, in 1989 Vietnam reformed the financing and delivery of health services by legalizing private medical practice, liberalizing the pharmaceutical industry and introducing user charges for public health facilities. These reforms turned Vietnam's near-universal, publicly funded healthcare system into a largely unregulated private–public mixed system. Over time, as state health budgets

Table 4.2 Health expenditure, 2002

Country	Total health expenditure (% of GDP)	Private expenditure as % of total expenditure	Out-of-pocket expenditure as % of private expenditure
Brunei	3.5	21.8	100.0
Cambodia	12.0	82.9	85.2
China	5.8	66.3	96.3
Indonesia	3.2	64.0	76.1
Japan	7.9	18.3	89.8
Laos	2.9	49.1	80.0
Malaysia	3.8	46.2	92.8
Myanmar	2.2	81.5	99.7
North Korea	4.6	23.4	100.0
Philippines	2.9	60.9	77.9
Singapore	4.3	69.1	97.3
South Korea	5.0	47.1	82.3
Thailand	4.4	30.3	75.8
Timor-Leste	9.7	36.1	51.9
Vietnam	5.2	70.8	87.6

Source: WHO, *World Health Report 2005: Make Every Mother and Child Count*, Geneva: World Health Organization, 2005, pp. 192–199.

decreased, and as public hospitals came to rely more heavily on user charges and insurance premiums to finance services, healthcare costs for low- and middle-income households increased substantially. By 1998, 80 per cent of health spending in Vietnam was being paid out-of-pocket, and an increased proportion of Vietnamese (approximately 40–60 per cent) presently rely on self-treatment or treatment outside of the healthcare system.[2]

In other countries, higher levels of insurance enable greater access to healthcare and thus potentially increase the chances of detecting disease outbreaks early. In the Philippines, less than half the population presently has insurance coverage, although the National Health Insurance Program is moving quickly towards its goal of providing health financing for most citizens.[3] Japanese citizens are covered comprehensively by either national medical insurance (for the self-employed) or social insurance (for employees).[4] And Thailand has had universal healthcare coverage since October 2001, financed by general tax revenue. Moreover, since 1972, the Thai government has enforced mandatory rural service for three years among new medicine, nursing, pharmacy and dentistry graduates. This has significantly improved access to quality medical services for the vast majority of Thailand's rural population.[5]

Disease surveillance

Directly related to the level of access to healthcare is a country's ability to detect and respond to disease outbreaks. The effectiveness of disease surveillance may be measured in terms of:

1   sensitivity – the capability to identify quickly and accurately an illness that is out of the ordinary; and
2   connectivity – the speed and accuracy with which this and related information is passed among medical professionals, public health entities and relevant international bodies.

In parts of East Asia, local factors could hinder the transparency required for a surveillance system that is both sensitive and connected. Most importantly, some countries in the region, having fragile economies, may be reluctant to admit the occurrence of outbreaks that would result in severe economic losses. With regard to H5N1 infection in poultry, for example, the OIE has documented delays as long as seven weeks between recognition and international reporting of outbreaks. One suggested explanation for this has been that the reporting authorities in some countries have dual and conflicting mandates both to report disease occurrences and to foster their country's export status for animal products.[6]

As international health agencies like the OIE lack enforcement powers, the reporting of diseases can only be voluntary. However, global electronic interconnectedness is gradually breaking down the traditional reluctance to do so. Of particular importance in defeating SARS in 2003 was the WHO Global Outbreak Alert and Response Network (GOARN). Under development since 1997, GOARN is a highly sensitive network of over 100 laboratories and disease-reporting systems, providing timely reports of infectious disease outbreaks. It is supported by a computer-driven tool for real-time gathering of disease intelligence, the Global Public Health Intelligence Network. This network continuously and systematically trawls websites, news wires, local online newspapers, public health email services and electronic discussion groups for rumours of outbreaks. This in turn allows the WHO to scan the world for news that might raise suspicions of an unusual disease event.

Global electronic disease surveillance systems provide for a high level of connectivity, although the sensitivity and effectiveness of such systems depends largely upon local surveillance backed up by adequate diagnostic laboratory capacity. Within East Asia, this is generally not a problem for wealthier countries. South Korea, for example, has a laboratory-based system for monitoring a number of diseases, including respiratory illnesses like influenza, and South Korean health professionals have since 1999 been able to access a disease reporting system via the Internet.[7] In the poorest parts of the region, however, national surveillance systems suffer from inadequate sensitivity and incomplete reporting of illness and outbreaks. In Laos, the National Center for Laboratory and Epidemiology monitors infectious diseases through a nationwide, hospital-based, active surveillance system. And, on a weekly basis, provincial surveillance units report the occurrence of infectious diseases in major hospitals and some district hospitals to the Ministry of Health. However, none of the national or provincial surveillance units have reliable

Internet access or email, and no system for laboratory-based surveillance exists in Laos. Nor is there such a system in neighbouring Cambodia.[8]

Disease surveillance is a vital means of knowing whether and to what extent an outbreak has occurred. Thereafter, the core mission of any outbreak response is to provide medical treatment to infected individuals. A key requirement for this is that national health systems are organized and equipped to cope with a sudden surge in patient demand.

Surge capacity

Even if a large proportion of a country's population was insured against the cost of medical treatment, and that country had in place a highly sensitive and well-connected disease surveillance system, there might not be enough health workers and hospital beds to accommodate a sudden influx of patients all demanding treatment at the same time. During an outbreak event, the human and physical resources of a national health system would be placed under greater pressure than usual. In early 2004, for example, Indonesia suffered an unusually severe outbreak of dengue (a disease caused by a mosquito-borne virus) that lasted until April of that year, causing more than 58,000 cases of illness and 650 deaths. In response, Indonesia's health authorities conducted intensive vector control activities and provided free hospital treatment to those dengue patients who could not afford to pay. By mid-March 2004, health workers exhausted by the number of patients had set up camp-beds in hospital corridors to cope with the crisis.[9] In addition to the treatment demands of the large number of people in fact stricken with an epidemic or pandemic disease, the health system would also face demands for medical attention from people with symptoms resembling those caused by the disease, as well as demands for prophylactic treatment from the 'worried well' (uninfected people fearful of contagion). From a disease surveillance and public health perspective, the danger is that these added demands would increase the chances of medical personnel overlooking some genuine victims of the outbreak.

Around the world, hospital staff and resources are usually stretched to the limit on day-to-day matters and generally cannot cope well with sudden small increases in patient numbers. In the face of outbreak threats of the kind analysed in this book, a key response is therefore to build a surge capacity into national health systems. Emergency plans would be needed in areas such as staff protection, patient triage on a mass scale, distributing and administering drugs and other therapy, and coordination with relevant national and international agencies. Specific measures to enhance surge capacity might include, for example:

- acquiring extra ventilators to support patients with pneumonia;
- building additional negative pressure rooms in hospitals to isolate patients infected with a contagious disease;

- putting in place back-up communication systems and power supplies; and
- providing diagnostic laboratories with the capacity to analyse an increased number of tissue samples from suspected outbreak victims – this is particularly important because diagnosis and research guide medical and public health response measures.

In addition to issues of capability, surge capacity is also about the willingness of health sector entities to provide emergency assistance. During the SARS outbreak in Taiwan, many hospitals refused to accept suspected SARS patients for fear that this would scare away other patients and thus reduce revenues.[10] This stands in contrast to Hong Kong, where there is presently a database of private-sector physicians willing to do volunteer work in government hospitals in the event of an influenza pandemic.[11] Another possibility along these lines is to create public health service reserves, akin to military reserves, to be called up in emergencies to perform low-level duties such as administering drugs and vaccines.[12] Lastly, depending on the extent to which an outbreak generates civil disorder, surge capacity may also need to extend beyond public health into the realms of emergency services, law enforcement and the supply of essential non-health services.

The case of China

On the issue of health resources in East Asia, China deserves special attention, not only because it is the largest and most populous country in the region, but also because this is where both SARS and H5N1 avian influenza first appeared. Conditions inside the country are such that more new diseases are likely to emerge from there in the future. In particular, farming practices in southern China provide an ideal environment for viruses to jump between species. According to the agricultural technique of 'polyculture', chickens are kept in cages suspended above pigs, which feed on the droppings. Fresh pig faeces are then used to fertilize fish ponds where ducks drink and defecate. And, in the midst of all this animal interaction, lives the Chinese farmer. In such circumstances, where viruses from pigs, people and birds have opportunities to exchange genes and mutate, the emergence of new influenza strains is a prime concern.

Another aspect of China's vulnerability to disease outbreaks is rapid urbanization, which is expanding the traditional role of cities as gateways for infections. China plans to increase its urban population from 37 per cent to 50 per cent by 2020, and it already has a floating population of around 120 to 130 million surplus labourers who are constantly moving between rural areas and the cities in search of work.[13] Internal migration on such a large scale has the potential to spark major epidemics as migrants introduce infectious diseases into new populations. And the influx of poor migrants into China's main cities brings overcrowding and sanitation problems, thus exacerbating the risk of disease transmission even further.

Against this microbial and demographic backdrop, the major factor exacerbating China's special vulnerability to infectious disease outbreaks is the inadequacy of its health system. During the era of a planned economy, China's communist regime developed one of the world's most comprehensive health systems, with healthcare in rural areas provided at the commune level through the Cooperative Medical System (CMS). From 1952 to 1982, infant mortality fell from 200 to 34 per 1,000 live births, and life expectancy increased from 35 to 68 years.[14] When the government later privatized the agricultural economy, however, communes were suddenly and completely dismantled. Without the CMS, Chinese peasants had no way to pool resources for healthcare expenses – in effect, privatization rendered 900 million rural citizens uninsured overnight. In 1978, out-of-pocket expenses accounted for 20 per cent of healthcare spending in China, as compared to 58 per cent in 2002, and only 29 per cent of Chinese presently have health insurance to cover the costs of care.[15] This is in circumstances where, in Beijing for example, the average cost of a stay at a state-run hospital is almost US$1,400 – a sum equal to half the annual salary of a typical city resident.[16]

The situation is worse in rural areas. After 20 years of uneven economic development, China's less-developed regions have far fewer hospitals, health professionals and medicines, and have less sanitation than the cities. China's rural citizens, who make up 70 per cent of the total population, presently use only 20 per cent of China's medical services and resources.[17] Moreover, according to a 2003 survey by the Chinese Ministry of Health, 79 per cent of rural citizens have no health insurance, and the prevalence of citizens who could not afford medical treatment rose from 32 per cent to 39 per cent in rural areas between 1993 and 2003.[18] Much of what people can pay instead goes to unlicensed and unqualified medical practitioners, or on unnecessary or inappropriate drugs sold by health clinics that rely heavily on pharmaceutical sales for funding. Lastly, under a system in which local doctors act on a fee-for-service basis, there is little incentive for them to visit remote villages to vaccinate children, preferring instead to concentrate on more lucrative work in the main towns and cities. Partly as a result of this, preventative health measures such as immunization have been ignored in many areas of China, leading to the resurgence of infectious diseases.[19]

On the whole, changes to the health system have significantly undermined China's ability to mount an effective, coordinated response to infectious disease outbreak threats. According to Yanzhong Huang, when SARS struck in 2003, China's efforts were compromised in three crucial respects:

1   lack of state funding – underfinanced local government healthcare systems did not have adequate resources to carry out SARS prevention and treatment;
2   lack of staff and facilities – among the 66,000 healthcare workers in Beijing, for example, less than 3,000 were familiar with respiratory diseases; and

3 inequalities in health resource distribution – the millions of peasant workers fleeing the cities to escape SARS threatened to spark a large-scale epidemic in rural areas where the health infrastructure is severely strained.[20]

Despite these structural handicaps, China nevertheless showed itself to be quite resourceful at an operational level during the SARS outbreak. Containment of the disease was facilitated by rapid training of medical staff in the use of protective equipment, the creation of fever clinics and improvements in patient management. The Chinese government was also able to supply 11 million surgical masks, gowns and gloves, and to quickly distribute 300 tonnes of disinfectant. And, after overcoming its initial reticence about publicly admitting to the existence of SARS, the government launched a massive media effort to alert its population to the risks of the disease.[21] In the immediate aftermath of the SARS outbreak, Beijing announced US$1.3 billion in new funding to the national health system for SARS prevention and the construction of quarantine facilities.[22] China has also since created a district-level, electronic system of disease reporting, and every district now has a designated infectious diseases hospital. Unfortunately, gaps in monitoring persist below the district level – as districts in China include hundreds of thousands of people, this means an outbreak could spread widely within a local population before it came to the attention of district authorities.[23]

The case of China well demonstrates the importance of strengthening healthcare and public health resources for the purpose of enhancing national outbreak response capacity. However, the responsibility for preventing or mitigating infectious diseases that may emerge from inside China does not rest with that country alone. The rest of the world, to which China is now highly connected in terms of travel and trade, is potentially at risk from new contagious diseases and thus has an interest in responding to outbreak threats through international action.

International action

In the face of microbial threats that transcend political borders, nationally focused outbreak-response efforts need to be supported and coordinated internationally. The final section of this chapter explores this requirement, first, by examining the notion of shared vulnerability to contagious diseases – bilateral assistance arrangements and existing regional organizations within East Asia potentially provide institutional architecture for collective security against such threats. Second, recent reforms of the WHO and the international legal framework in which it operates could greatly enhance its ability to lead and coordinate outbreak-response efforts. Lastly, there is increasing scope for naturally occurring disease threats to be addressed through the Biological Weapons Convention.

Shared vulnerability

In an age of international air travel, which makes all countries vulnerable to new contagious diseases, there is a strong collective security imperative behind international action to address outbreak threats. A disease outbreak is more likely to acquire international significance if it occurs in a place where there is insufficient national capacity to:

1   recognize quickly the occurrence and extent of the outbreak;
2   deploy trained personnel to investigate and confirm reports of illness;
3   identify the disease's causative agent in the laboratory; and
4   implement effective interventions to contain the spread of disease.

Thus, rather than waiting for a disease that is out of control in such a country to spread beyond its borders, unaffected countries can potentially protect themselves by providing timely assistance at the outbreak's source.

In the face of specific outbreak threats, wealthier countries in East Asia have provided bilateral assistance on a short-term basis. For example, in May 2003, Japan granted China 1.5 billion yen in emergency aid to deal with SARS and extended separate aid grants to Beijing (ten million yen) and Shanghai (17 million yen). Japan also sent disaster relief teams to Vietnam (March 2003) and China (May 2003) to provide practical assistance with SARS countermeasures. In February 2004, to counter the threat posed by H5N1 avian influenza, Japan provided medicines worth 20 million yen to Vietnam. The following month, Japanese experts were sent to Thailand, Cambodia, Laos and Myanmar, with Laos also receiving diagnosis equipment worth US$50,000.[24] In addition, from outside the region, Australia in 2005 donated 50,000 doses of Tamiflu to Indonesia and committed to spend A$100 million over four years helping countries in the region resist H5N1.[25] In the same year, US President George W. Bush announced an influenza assistance package worth US$251 million 'to help our foreign partners [in East Asia] train local medical personnel, expand their surveillance and testing capacity, draw up preparedness plans, and take other vital actions to detect and contain outbreaks'.[26]

Security against outbreak threats in the long term, however, requires sustained efforts to enhance the national health systems of developing countries. Financial contributions would be more than simple acts of charity – rather, wealthy donor countries would be helping to pay for systems that would bring great health and security benefits to them as well. Specifically, well-resourced countries could protect themselves against outbreak threats of international proportions by helping developing countries to create a strong public health infrastructure, educating local health professionals and sponsoring appropriate measures to enable timely identification and control of infectious diseases.

Such assistance has already been granted to countries in East Asia by donors outside the region. Australia, for example, has stated that it is in that country's own best interests to be a major player in regional surveillance and to ensure that the mechanisms used for this purpose are the best available. This is essentially because detecting and responding to overseas outbreaks relieves the Australian health system of infectious disease casualties that might otherwise arrive undetected in Australia. To this end, Australia deploys epidemiologists and microbiologists throughout East Asia to engage in surveillance, laboratory diagnosis and outbreak investigation.[27] The United States too has made some valuable contributions to health in the region, such as the opening in May 2004 of the Regional Emerging Diseases Intervention (REDI) Centre in Singapore. Jointly established by the US and Singapore governments, REDI is intended to strengthen infectious disease surveillance and outbreak response capabilities through research and training.[28]

Prior to this, in October 2001, the US government launched its first International Emerging Infections Program (IEIP) in Thailand. This programme maintains relations with medical research institutes, local universities, the Thai Field Epidemiology Training Program, US military laboratories, and WHO country and regional offices. Its purpose is to strengthen national public health capacity and provide practical training in laboratory science, epidemiology and public health administration. By bringing advanced laboratory diagnostic capability to a field investigation, the IEIP strengthens Thailand's existing capacity for outbreak investigation, especially with regard to infectious diseases previously unknown to medical science. During the 2003 SARS outbreak, for example, US and Thai epidemiologists worked together to set up mobile evaluation and training teams with checklists and information packs on infection control measures. The IEIP also assisted the regional response to SARS by sending teams to meet urgent requests for assistance from Taiwan, Laos, Hong Kong, China and Singapore.[29]

Within East Asia itself, a consciousness of shared vulnerability may lead to greater cooperation against outbreak threats through existing regional organizations. The ASEAN and ASEAN+3 groupings, for example, have already demonstrated their ability to respond effectively to SARS, and the issue of H5N1 is presently being addressed via the security-oriented ASEAN Regional Forum (ARF). A meeting of the ARF Inter-Sessional Support Group on Confidence-Building Measures in April 2004 identified infectious diseases as posing a serious challenge and called for closer regional cooperation and mutual support, including capacity building, information sharing and intelligence exchange among ARF participants.[30] And at the twelfth ARF Meeting in July 2005, the ministers in attendance specifically acknowledged the importance of robust disease surveillance and timely reporting of human H5N1 cases, and the need for countries to develop national pandemic influenza preparedness plans.[31]

Another possible forum for addressing outbreak threats is the Asia-Pacific Economic Cooperation (APEC) group of countries which, among other measures, has established an emerging infectious diseases network, APEC

EINet, to facilitate Internet-based information sharing throughout the region.[32] Importantly, international consultations under APEC auspices are more inclusive because, unlike ASEAN, the grouping formally includes Australia, Taiwan and the United States. At the November 2005 APEC Meeting in South Korea, the economic leaders endorsed the APEC Initiative on Preparing For and Mitigating an Influenza Pandemic, which commits APEC economies to

> strengthening cooperation and technical assistance among APEC economies to limit avian influenza at its source and prevent human outbreaks; developing a list of available and funded regional experts and capabilities for responding rapidly to pandemic influenza in its early stages; testing pandemic preparedness, beginning with a desk-top simulation exercise in early 2006 to test regional responses and communication networks; enhancing public and business outreach and risk communication; and exchanging information on border screening procedures and controls to increase transparency and to reduce risk to trade and travellers.[33]

It remains to be seen, however, how effective an APEC-driven cooperative response to outbreak threats would be. The principal concern is that APEC as a whole has lately appeared somewhat moribund, not least because the East Asian Summit has emerged as a competitor organization in the region. In any case, it is most likely that the role of East Asian regional organizations in preventing or responding to outbreaks would be secondary to that of the WHO. This institution has greater scientific authority and a clearer public health mission than groupings like ASEAN and APEC. And, as a consequence of recent reforms to the legal framework in which it operates, the WHO is soon to acquire greater powers and responsibilities.

Reform of the World Health Organization

The WHO has long been regarded as lacking the resources and authority to deal effectively with health problems around the world. From June 2007, however, when recent comprehensive revisions of the International Health Regulations (IHR) come into effect, the organization is likely to have a greatly enhanced capacity to respond to outbreak threats. The IHR govern the roles of the WHO and its member states in identifying and responding to public health emergencies and sharing information about them. Their purpose is to ensure maximum protection of people against the international spread of diseases, while minimizing interference with world travel and trade. At the time the disease that became known as SARS first emerged in China, the IHR required WHO member states to promptly report outbreaks of cholera, plague and yellow fever that occurred in their territory. As such, although China's reluctance in early 2003 to cooperate with the WHO and other governments may have made the public health threat from SARS worse, its behaviour did not contravene international law. The SARS outbreak thus made conspicuous the deficiencies of the existing system of international health governance, and the spectre of pandemic influenza that emerged shortly afterwards increased further the impetus to reform that system.

On 23 May 2005, after a decade of deliberation, the fifty-eighth World Health Assembly (comprising the 192 member states of the WHO) adopted new IHR setting out how to respond to international disease threats. Under the revised regulations, the WHO has broader powers, and countries have greater obligations, to detect and respond to public health emergencies of international concern.[34] For the purposes of this chapter, the four most important areas of reform are:

1   strengthening national health system capacity;
2   disease reporting;
3   the use of non-official information; and
4   cooperation between the sectors responsible for human and animal health.

First, regarding national health system capacity, the new IHR designate the following as the core components of a country's preparedness to detect and respond to infectious disease threats: early warning and routine surveillance systems; epidemiological and outbreak investigation skills; laboratory expertise; information and communication technologies; and management systems. It is widely accepted that uniformly strong national public health systems that can rapidly detect and respond to health threats at their source are vital for preventing local infectious disease crises from becoming global. Accordingly, the new IHR give WHO member states two years to assess their capabilities to identify, verify and respond to health emergencies, and five years to develop such capabilities. Nevertheless, implementing this reform is likely to entail considerable expense, and many developing countries are already struggling to establish and maintain the public health infrastructure necessary to care for their populations. Cambodia, for example, already spends 12 per cent of its GDP on health (see Table 4.2). Although the new IHR impose a duty on the WHO to support capacity-building at the national level, much will depend on wealthy countries voluntarily providing financial and technical assistance.

Second, under the revised system of outbreak notification, there remains a list of diseases whose occurrence must be reported to the WHO – this includes SARS and human influenza caused by a new viral subtype. In addition, the new IHR provide four criteria to assist states in deciding whether the WHO needs to know about other disease events:

1   is the public health impact of the event serious?
2   is the event unusual or unexpected?

3   is there a significant risk of international spread?
4   is there a significant risk of international restrictions to travel and trade?

Any event meeting more than one of the four criteria must be reported, and countries are required to communicate detailed public health information during an outbreak, including case definitions, laboratory results, number of cases and deaths, and conditions affecting the spread of the disease.

According to Lawrence Gostin, a possible drawback of this reform is that, because the old reporting requirements were more straightforward by comparison, it could lead some countries to throw up their hands in confusion and lower their national disease surveillance standards. To counter this, Gostin argues, the WHO would need to provide detailed advice and assistance, particularly about diseases, conditions and events that are notifiable.[35] On the other hand, an important new incentive for countries to report outbreaks is the establishment, under the revised IHR, of expert panels to review the risks to international public health and recommend evidence-based control measures. This is a partial remedy to the situation under the old regulations in which some countries were reluctant to report disease outbreaks because unaffected countries tended to apply travel and trade restrictions disproportionate to the true risks of the disease.

The third major reform of the IHR is a standing authorization for the WHO to use a range of sources of intelligence to raise an alarm and begin a process of verification with countries that have not voluntarily reported significant outbreak events. On this point, it is important to note that informal Internet discussion groups such as FluNet and ProMED are often the first to identify a significant percentage of outbreaks. Under the new IHR, if the WHO obtains credible evidence that a public health event of international importance has occurred, and the affected country fails to disclose this officially or to cooperate, the organization is authorized to release whatever relevant information is required to protect global public health. The background to this reform is that the use of non-official information proved vital in combating the SARS outbreak, especially in China where official advice to, and cooperation with, the WHO were not quickly forthcoming. During the early part of the outbreak, the WHO independently issued a global alert, and made geographically-specific travel recommendations, all without express authorization under the WHO Constitution, the IHR or from the states directly affected. But member states acquiesced to such actions by the WHO at the time and then formally directed its Director General to issue similar alerts in the future when necessary.[36] The revised IHR have therefore enshrined in international law what had already become an accepted WHO practice.

Lastly, the new IHR expressly require the WHO to cooperate and coordinate its activities with the FAO and the OIE. Cooperation and exchange of information between the public health and veterinary sectors are important because many disease outbreaks of international concern are the result of zoonosis. The animal origins of SARS and H5N1 influenza have generated a new imperative for international organizations, which have little or no tradition of cooperation, to join forces. Examples of this include: the recent formation of the OIE–FAO Network of Expertise on Avian Influenza, which works in collaboration with the WHO Global Influenza Network; the Global Strategy for the Progressive Control of Highly Pathogenic Avian Influenza, jointly written by the FAO, OIE and the WHO; and the FAO–OIE–WHO Consultation on Avian Influenza and Human Health, which has proposed risk-reduction measures for producing, marketing and living with animals in Asia.[37]

The WHO, acting within the legal framework of the IHR, is an institution primarily concerned with infectious disease outbreaks of natural origin. However, it has been the case in the past that a disease outbreak caused by the deliberate dissemination of pathogenic micro-organisms can be difficult to distinguish from a naturally occurring outbreak. From the perspective of the WHO, however, a disease outbreak of whatever origin is still a public health problem requiring a public health solution. Accordingly, part of the WHO's role is also to advise countries on preparedness for and responses to the use of BW.[38] This brings the organization alongside another international institution that aims to eliminate infectious disease threats to countries around the world – the Biological Weapons Convention (BWC). In turn, the BWC regime, which is discussed further in later chapters of this book, offers opportunities to address many of the public health challenges with which the WHO is mainly concerned.

The Biological Weapons Convention

The BWC is a universal disarmament treaty that came into force in 1975. Although primarily aimed at addressing the problem of BW, it also provides scope to address outbreak threats of natural origin. This is a consequence of the fact that, from a response perspective, there are extensive synergies and crossovers between these two disease-based security challenges. For example, as WHO representative David Heymann testified to the US Senate Foreign Relations Committee in 2001: 'the epidemiological techniques needed to investigate deliberate and natural outbreaks are the same.'[39] Overlapping security and public health concerns were behind a collaboration in 2003 between US and Thai biologists to research *Burkholderia pseudomallei* – a common bacterium in Thailand that causes the disease melioidosis, against which there is no vaccine. Although around 5,000 Thais die each year from the disease, the US interest was driven mainly by fears that *B. pseudomallei* could be used in a biological attack.[40]

With regard to the BWC itself, the substantial overlap between deliberate and natural disease threats was most clearly demonstrated in the new negotiating process that emerged from the Fifth BWC Review Conference in 2002. Specifically, at their 2004 meeting in Geneva, BWC member states had a mandate to 'discuss, and promote common understanding and effective action' on 'strengthening and broadening national and international institutional efforts and existing mechanisms for the surveillance, detection, diagnosis and combating of infectious diseases affecting humans, animals, and plants'.[41] At the conclusion of this meeting, in the course of which the Australian ambassador Michael Smith had urged countries 'to consider disease control as a mainstream security issue not just a matter of health',[42] the BWC member states agreed on the value of:

a   Supporting the existing networks of relevant international organisations for the surveillance, detection, diagnosis and combating of infectious diseases and acting to strengthen the WHO, FAO and OIE programmes, within their mandates, for the continued development and strengthening of, and research into, rapid, effective and reliable activities for the surveillance, detection, diagnosis and combating of infectious diseases, including in cases of emergencies of international concern;

b   Improving, wherever possible, national and regional disease surveillance capabilities, and, if in a position to do so, assisting and encouraging, with the necessary agreement, other States Parties to do the same;

c   Working to improve communication on disease surveillance, including with the WHO, FAO and OIE, and among States Parties.[43]

Although synergies between public health and security can be used to good effect, it is nevertheless important to note that the overlaps between concerns about BW and natural disease threats can occasionally generate difficulties. In early 2004, for example, Hong Kong-based virologist Guan Yi was researching H5N1 avian influenza that had infected poultry in Japan. Obtaining virus samples from Japan ran into trouble because both the Hong Kong and Japanese governments, concerned about BW threats, had designated H5N1 as a biological agent requiring special handling. The Hong Kong permit Guan needed to import samples was valid for one week only, whereas Japan's National Institute for Infectious Diseases was not able to obtain export approval that quickly.[44] In effect, concern about the possibility of deliberate disease was stifling responses to a clear and present infectious disease threat of natural origin. Nevertheless, as will be discussed in Part III of this book, laboratory research on pathogenic micro-organisms carries its own set of security risks.

Conclusion

Rallying around states, which are the principal providers of health services, is the key to responding to actual and potential outbreak events. This chapter has accordingly examined the importance of national health resources, measured in terms of access to care, disease surveillance and health system surge capacity. Within the East Asian region, the poorest developing countries (for example, Cambodia, Laos and Myanmar) are likely to be particularly vulnerable to outbreaks occurring in their territory because of a paucity of health resources. Countries such as China may be vulnerable because health resources are allocated so unevenly as to open up gaps in outbreak response capacity.

For the purposes of outbreak prevention and response, although national capacity is the primary focus, the profoundly international nature of microbial threats that transcend political borders demands cooperative action. The security imperative for such action is shared vulnerability in a highly connected world – in circumstances where a disease like pandemic influenza was transmitted easily between people, transmission between countries would be facilitated by international air travel. For wealthy countries that may be geographically removed from the origin of an outbreak, time and space are today of little significance. For this reason, such countries have an interest in enhancing outbreak response capabilities in the developing world. The primary mechanism for international assistance and cooperation is the WHO, the powers of which are likely to increase under new IHR. In addition, within the context of East Asia, there may be scope to address infectious disease threats through existing regional organizations like ASEAN and APEC. Lastly, the BWC could play an important role in addressing naturally occurring outbreak threats as well as the threat of deliberate disease. This institutional incursion into public health by a treaty ostensibly about arms control is but one example of the extent to which, from a security perspective, natural plagues are a challenge closely akin to biological weapons.

Part II
Biological weapons

5   The science and history of deliberate disease

This chapter introduces the problem of biological weapons (BW) by placing it in scientific and historical context. At the outset, it is vital to note that BW threats are diverse in their effects and scale; they are not simply 'weapons of mass destruction' (WMD). The first section examines the scientific and technical aspects of biological agents and their means of delivery. These are important considerations for a state in choosing whether to acquire and/or maintain a BW capability. This is followed by a section that assesses the military value of such a capability in two dimensions – the tactical utility of BW and their strategic significance. The final section surveys the historical record of modern BW use, actual and alleged, in East Asia. This covers the period from the 1930s and Imperial Japan's biological warfare programme to present-day suspicions that North Korea and China possess BW.

Science and technology

To understand and respond to the problem of BW, a vital first step is to rescue it from the awkward rubric of 'WMD'. Strictly speaking, only nuclear weapons cause mass destruction. Chemical and biological weapons attack living tissue but do not destroy non-animate objects, and the number of casualties they cause is highly dependent on the choice of agent and the conditions under which it is disseminated. The linguistic device of grouping together under one term weapons that are technically vastly different carries the risk that the uniqueness of each may be overlooked by policy-makers. Nuclear, biological and chemical weapons differ greatly in terms of ease of production, efficiency and predictability, challenges for deterrence, and effective response measures. Scientific differences translate into tactical and strategic ones, such that analogizing between the three purported categories of WMD is largely inappropriate.

For at least two reasons, it is necessary to avoid approaching BW as solely a WMD issue. First, in contrast to nuclear weapons, the ability to cause mass casualties is a potential property of BW rather than an inherent one. The common tendency to classify BW as WMD is misleading because the extent of harm resulting from their use is highly dependent on: the type and quantity of agent released; the means by which it is delivered; the environmental conditions at the target; and whether and how soon medical intervention is available. Repeated references to BW as a mass-casualty problem serve to focus attention on the worst-case end of the threat spectrum, and such references usually occur without the reassurance that mass casualties are also the least likely outcome of BW use.

Second, and most importantly, defending against a biological attack has more in common with confronting emerging infectious disease threats of natural origin than preparation for a nuclear or chemical attack. In terms of likely consequences, a natural outbreak of a deadly, contagious disease would, like a biological attack, be unannounced and the disease would spread undetected for some time before being identified and treated. Questions would then arise about how to cope with an unfamiliar pathogenic micro-organism. Whether a disease outbreak is natural or deliberate, the public health arena is where the main struggle would take place. In this context, it is more appropriate to regard BW less as 'weapons' and more as one part of a spectrum of disease-based security challenges.

To illustrate how BW are more than just a WMD threat, the following sections examine biological agents and their means of delivery. BW effects are diverse in nature and scale, and achieving mass casualties can be difficult.

Biological agents

Biological agents are infectious micro-organisms (bacteria, viruses, fungi and rickettsia) that reproduce within the host to cause an incapacitating or fatal illness. A particular micro-organism can cause serious disease and yet be unsuitable for a biological attack. For example, the virus (HIV) that causes AIDS would not be an effective BW agent because its average incubation period of ten years is too slow to have any tactical or strategic value. Also, the virus cannot be transmitted through the air. Assuming a biological agent reaches and infects its target, the amount of resulting human damage depends upon the choice of agent and its virulence, whether the disease it causes is contagious and how easily it can be treated. The following examples illustrate the diversity of BW challenges.

Bacillus anthracis is a spore-forming bacterium that causes pulmonary anthrax if it infects the lungs. Victims suffer fever, severe breathing difficulties, shock, pneumonia and death within days of exposure. A large proportion of people deliberately infected with *B. anthracis* are likely to die; however, the effects of an anthrax attack will be limited because the disease is generally not contagious and can be treated with antibiotics. However, a person might not know he or she has been infected – this is a problem because anthrax infection needs to be treated quickly. Rather, that person might interpret their symptoms (cough, chest pains, aches and fever) as a bad cold. Delaying antibiotic treatment even by hours may substantially lessen a patient's chances of survival.[1]

Yersinia pestis is the bacterium that causes plague. It is typically transmitted by flea bites (bubonic plague) but if it infects the lungs, the disease can transmit through the air from person to person. Death is caused by respiratory and circulatory collapse from septic shock. Untreated pneumonic plague is 100 per cent fatal. Vaccination against plague during an epidemic would not be very effective as immunity takes a month to build up. And, although a plague sufferer can be treated successfully with antibiotics, fatality rates remain high if treatment does not commence within 24 hours of the onset of symptoms.[2]

Variola major virus causes smallpox, a highly contagious disease that cannot usually be treated after infection. It kills around 30 per cent of those it infects. After the end of the Cold War, it emerged that the Soviet Union had, from as early as the 1970s, grown and stockpiled tons of *variola* as part of its secret BW programme. This gave rise to fears that some of this vast quantity might have been stolen and possibly sold on by former Soviet scientists. Nevertheless, *variola* cannot be said to be a readily available biological agent. Smallpox was declared eradicated from nature in 1980, whereas all the above agents exist in the natural environment or as reference strains in many laboratories. On the other hand, because routine vaccination in most countries ceased well before the eradication of smallpox, almost the entire world's population presently has little or no immunity. At present, the only treatment available to a smallpox patient would be supportive care and antibiotics to prevent secondary infection. There are currently no antiviral drugs effective against smallpox, although vaccination administered within a few days of exposure may prevent or mitigate the disease.[3]

Preparation and delivery

Once a biological agent has been selected to cause a particular effect, it must be prepared in a form that can readily infect humans and then delivered efficiently to its target. For achieving mass casualties, weaponization requirements differ according to the nature of the agent to be used. If a perpetrator chooses a non-contagious disease like anthrax, a sophisticated delivery system is required for dispersing the agent over a large area – every victim has to come into direct contact with the agent. With a contagious disease like pneumonic plague, however, delivery of the causative agent (*Y. pestis*) need not be so efficient or wide-scale. It might only be necessary to directly infect a small number of people, after which the initial victims would themselves spread the disease to others.

In 1970, the WHO estimated 250,000 casualties following the aircraft release of 50 kg of anthrax over an urban population of five million. Of these, 100,000 would die if left untreated.[4] And, in 1993, the US Congress Office of Technology Assessment estimated that the aerosolized release of 100 kg of anthrax upwind of the Washington, DC area would result in 130,000–3,000,000 deaths – achieving a lethality exceeding that of a nuclear weapon.[5] It is important to note, however, that neither of these analyses referred to empirical data. Indeed, for national security reasons, there is no unclassified data available generally on human exposure to deliberate, large-scale aerosol releases of biological agents. The following discussion of requirements for effective agent preparation and delivery is therefore necessarily based on scientific principles rather than historical experience.

When exposed to environmental stresses, *B. anthracis* bacteria form rugged spores resilient during processing and dissemination. Other biological agents are less hardy. For example, *Y. pestis* bacteria are non-spore-forming and thus more vulnerable to environmental factors, and viruses in general are more susceptible to ultraviolet light. Cold, clear nights or early in the morning are times when the atmospheric conditions are most suitable for effective delivery of biological agents. However, in the absence of perfect release conditions, and to reduce the degradation of agents by stresses such as desiccation, sunlight, freezing, as well as mechanical dissemination, it is necessary to enhance agent stability. One stabilization method is lyophilization – rapid freezing and subsequent dehydration under a high vacuum. Another method is microencapsulation, which emulates natural spore formation by coating droplets of a selected size with a thin coat of protective material.[6]

Preparation of a quantity of biological agent also requires that it consist of particles 1–5 microns in diameter (1 micron equals one-millionth of a metre). This allows the agent to travel to the alveolar spaces of the lungs where gas exchange in and out of the bloodstream occurs. Particles less than 1 micron in diameter are mostly exhaled without being retained in the deep lung tissue. And large particles, or small ones clumped together, tend to drop straight to the ground rather than stay suspended in the air ready for inhalation. The addition of anti-agglomerants such as silica helps to prevent the clumping of freeze-dried biological agents that have been milled into a fine powder. Particle clumping during dissemination can also be reduced by electrostatic charging of microcapsulated particles.[7] Depending on the biological agent used, particles of a suitable size would still need to be inhaled in sufficient quantities to cause illness and/or death. A 1960 study of environmental exposure at a US goat-hair mill found that workers inhaled up to 510 *B. anthracis* particles of at least 5 microns in diameter per person per eight-hour shift without any cases of inhalation anthrax occurring.[8]

For BW purposes, infecting members of a target population with the number of micro-organisms necessary to cause disease depends upon how efficiently they are delivered. Efficiency can be reduced by the target environment and/or by the chosen means of dissemination. For example, according to US tests, the stress from explosive dissemination can reduce the efficiency of biological agents to around 5 per cent.[9] And, if delivering BW over hilly or city terrain, atmospheric turbulence impedes even distribution and increases vertical dilution of the agent, thus reducing casualties.[10] As regards contamination of food or drinking water with biological agents, the consensus in the expert literature on BW appears to be that this would likely not succeed in causing many casualties. Dilution, chlorination and filtration work against water-borne agents, and cooking, pasteurization and other routine food safety precautions are also generally sufficient to kill pathogenic bacteria.[11] Nevertheless, deliberate contamination of non-processed food has occurred in the past. For example, in 1984, members of the US-based Rajneesh cult who sprinkled salmonella bacteria over salad bars in Oregon succeeded in sickening 751 people.[12] Generally speaking, however, the most efficient mode of entry for pathogenic micro-organisms is via the lungs.

Aerosol delivery of biological agents allows for the control of particle size and density to protect against environmental degradation and to maximize inhalation of particles by the target population. As aerosols are tasteless, odourless and invisible, they are highly suitable for clandestine delivery. The former Soviet Union reportedly had plans for the conspicuous delivery of smallpox virus loaded into intercontinental ballistic missiles (ICBMs),[13] even though these would likely be an inefficient and probably ineffective means of BW delivery. Live biological agents inside an ICBM warhead would have to survive the stresses of space flight and atmospheric re-entry. And because re-entry speed is so high, it would be difficult to distribute the agent in a diffuse cloud or with sufficient precision to ensure its release at a suitable altitude. A cloud of BW agent must be released below an atmospheric shear layer or it will disperse before reaching the ground – most shear layers occur at around 500 feet above ground level.[14] By the same reasoning, however, a cruise missile is potentially a highly effective means of BW delivery. Using an aerosol sprayer embedded in its wings and built-in meteorological sensors coupled to the guidance and control computer, a cruise missile could adjust its flight profile and release a quantity of biological agent tailored to the local topography, meteorological conditions and shape of the target, thus maximizing the potential for casualties.[15] The missile would need to be designed to release the agent outside of the aerodynamically disturbed flow field around the vehicle, and it would have to travel at below supersonic speed lest the airstream destroy the agent by heating or shock.[16]

The science and technology underlying BW, the diversity of biological agents and their effects, and the challenges of delivering them efficiently are factors relevant to the military value of deliberate disease. The next section explores why a state might choose to acquire and/or maintain a BW capability, and assesses the utility of such weapons at the tactical and strategic levels.

Why choose biological weapons?

On 25 November 1969, US President Richard Nixon declared:

> Biological weapons have massive unpredictable and potentially uncontrollable consequences. They may produce global epidemics and impair the health of future generations. I have therefore decided that the US shall renounce the use of lethal biological agents and weapons, and all other methods of biological warfare.[17]

Nixon's decision strengthened the international norm against BW as vile instruments of war to be eschewed by civilized nations, but it was also a pragmatic step to discard a category of weapons thought to be of limited military utility. Almost 40 years later, advances in biotechnology notwithstanding, uncertainties regarding the value of a BW programme remain relevant to whether a state would want to acquire such a capability in the first place. The following sections assess the advantages and disadvantages of BW as tactical weapons in war and as a strategic deterrent. Tactical capabilities are those directed towards engaging an adversary's front line military forces, immediate reinforcements, or supply lines. A strategic capability is aimed at an adversary's military infrastructure, economic base and/or civilian population that enable it to wage war.

Tactical utility

The caveat on arguments about the tactical utility of BW is that they stem mostly from theory and conjecture rather than recent experience. There has not been a confirmed incident of BW use in modern warfare since the Second World War. And the two most recent conflicts in which BW have been cited as a concern (the 1991 Gulf War and the 2003 Iraq War) illustrate the historical precedent of *not* using such weapons. An explanation for non-use in 2003, for example, might be that Iraq was not able to deploy BW at the crucial time. However, there are at least two other possible explanations:

1   that Iraq did not in fact possess BW before and during the invasion by US-led forces; or
2   that it was never part of Iraqi battle plans to use BW – rather, such weapons (if an adversary could be convinced they existed) were intended purely as a strategic deterrent. Thus, in the context of the Iraq War, BW were unable to be used, non-existent or not intended to be used.

Despite the paucity of empirical information regarding the tactical utility of BW, it is possible nevertheless to imagine certain identifiable advantages and disadvantages to using BW in war. One advantage is that, provided the enemy lacks effective detection and protection gear, the use of BW can have a devastating psychological impact, undermining the morale of troops and impairing their combat functions. Even forcing the enemy into protective equipment has advantages because this is a cumbersome measure that degrades military performance and slows down combat operations. Away from the front line, BW could be targeted at air bases, ships, ports, command centres and other supportive infrastructure in order to undermine an enemy's ability to mobilize and supply its troops in the field. Disadvantages undermining the military utility of BW include: the potential instability of agents after dissemination; vulnerability to meteorological factors that might kill biological agents in the air or carry them off target; the lengthy incubation period between a target's exposure to BW agents and the onset of disease; and the potential unpredictability of the effects of a BW attack.[18] Regarding the last point, however, Malcolm Dando has warned that there are now fewer uncertainties when considering the potential effectiveness of BW. As a result of an increased capacity for computer modelling, for example, some countries now have a far greater understanding of the atmospheric and weather conditions required for an optimal BW attack. In addition, some countries now have an extensive understanding of how inhaled aerosols behave inside the human lung.[19]

Assessing the tactical utility of BW is difficult without empirical data. However, for the present at least, it seems the fundamental disadvantages of using BW probably outweigh the value of their indirect and probably non-decisive effect on the outcome of war. The next section assesses whether BW could *prevent* war in a manner comparable to nuclear deterrence.

Strategic value

Some countries threatened by nuclear-armed adversaries might suppose BW provide rough strategic parity because of the theoretical potential for high casualties from a biological attack. A basic BW capability is much more affordable than a nuclear programme, and biological agents properly prepared and delivered under ideal conditions could inflict human damage to an extent comparable to a nuclear strike. According to Susan Martin, even the small probability of successful retaliation using BW can deter an attack. As a consequence, she argues, the spread of this attractive option among poorer countries could lead to a 'biological revolution' comparable to the post-Second World War nuclear revolution that would provide even weak states with the ability to deter threats to their vital interests.[20] However, Martin probably overstates the utility of BW as a strategic deterrent. The so-called 'poor man's atomic bomb' is in fact a poor substitute. Unless and until BW have the same demonstrable and assured destructive power as nuclear weapons, it is inappropriate to regard them as having a comparable deterrent value. For the purpose of strategic calculations, the vital difference is the uncertainty that surrounds the likely effects of a biological attack and the very existence of BW programmes. By contrast, the destructive power of nuclear weapons can be tested conspicuously.

The idea of BW-based strategic deterrence is problematic, first, because of the challenge of effective agent delivery. Considerations of the strategic reach of BW often involve analogies to nuclear weapons, particularly on the issue of long-range delivery to enemy cities using ICBMs or aircraft. However, the need for favourable weather conditions at the target means a BW state is restricted in choosing when and where to launch a retaliatory strike. And with ballistic missile delivery, the great technical challenge is to preserve the stability and virulence of biological agents during the stress of space flight and the heat encountered when a warhead re-enters the atmosphere. A second major problem is that the secrecy surrounding BW programmes makes them an unreliable deterrent. As these weapons are banned categorically under international law, countries in possession of them could not publicly proclaim their existence without suffering political opprobrium. Such countries must necessarily rely, paradoxically, on an undeclared deterrent capability. This is the opposite of how deterrence generally works in the nuclear realm. In stark contrast to the secrecy surrounding BW, nuclear status is institutionalized (under the 1968 Nuclear Non-proliferation Treaty), nuclear tests have been conducted openly in the hope of gaining political leverage (India and Pakistan) and nuclear ambitions have been flaunted for strategic bargaining purposes (North Korea and Iran).[21] Compared to the relatively brazen world of nuclear deterrence, a BW-based deterrent capability would involve far greater uncertainty. Enhancing the credibility of a state's deterrent threat would necessarily entail revealing at least some information about the nature of its BW capabilities. However, the revelation of details such as types of biological agents to be used could reduce the effectiveness of a threatened BW strike by compromising the element of surprise and allowing the defender to take appropriate pharmaceutical and public health countermeasures.[22] The effects of a nuclear attack cannot be mitigated, but the damage from a BW attack can be reduced if effective medical treatment for victims is available.

Biological weapons and East Asia

The tactical and strategic shortcomings of BW notwithstanding, various countries have from time to time regarded such weapons as worthwhile. East Asia was the scene for BW use, actual and alleged, at various times during the last century and suspicions about BW possession persist in the region to this day. Commencing in the 1930s, the Imperial Japanese Army's BW programme, deployed against China before and during the Second World War, was the largest ever example of the systematic use of, and experimentation with, biological agents for military purposes. After the United States was victorious in the war, it closed a deal with ex-Japanese Army scientists to acquire BW data. The United States itself was soon afterwards accused by China and North Korea of using BW during the Korean War and, for the past 50 years, this allegation has been extremely difficult to resolve. This is partly attributable to the absence of publicly available official papers that would confirm the deployment of BW in the Korean theatre by the United States. But it is also a consequence of the difficulty, especially in wartime, of distinguishing between naturally and deliberately caused outbreaks of infectious disease. Evidentiary difficulties arose, for example, when an international human rights organization accused the Myanmar government of using BW against minority peoples in the early 1990s. And, to this day, uncertainty surrounds allegations that North Korea and China are BW states.

Unit 731: Imperial Japan and biological warfare

Imperial Japan ran a BW programme from 1932 to 1945, the development of which was led by Lieutenant General Shiro Ishii, head of the Kwantung Army's Unit 731. From the time of the Japanese occupation of parts of China through to the end of the Second World War, Unit 731 experimented on Chinese civilians and Allied prisoners of war with various biological agents, including those that cause plague, cholera and haemorrhagic fever. Unit 731 consisted of a laboratory complex of 150 buildings and five satellite camps. The main BW research compound was at Ping Fan, south of the Manchurian city of Harbin. It covered an area of six square kilometres and employed 3,000 Japanese doctors, technicians and soldiers.[23] Ishii regarded Manchuria as the ideal place for BW research because his unit's work could be camouflaged by the poor sanitary conditions of the area, where the spread of deadly infectious diseases was quite common. For example, Manchuria had previously been afflicted by cholera in 1919 and by pneumonic plague in 1910–1911, 1920–1921 and 1927.[24]

Plague held a particular fascination for Ishii. As the disease was endemic in China, the results of deliberate attacks with *Y. pestis* bacteria could, if carried out covertly, be mistaken for natural plague outbreaks. The question then was how to deliver the agent effectively. When the Japanese tried dropping plague-filled bombs from aircraft, the explosion killed the bacteria. After experimentation, they found that a more effective delivery method was to cover a target area with plague-infected fleas.[25] Ishii's great personal enthusiasm for this method led him to develop a porcelain bomb as a delivery system. These bombs carried grain to attract rats which were bitten by the infected fleas, thereby transmitting plague bacteria to human populations via vectors.[26] It had been Ishii's idea that a fragile porcelain bomb would be easier to detonate, require less explosive, cause less heat, and thus be much safer for the infected fleas inside. A 25 kg bomb, called the *Uji*, was filled with fleas and sand. Supplied with oxygen so the fleas would withstand high altitudes, the *Uji* could be dropped from beyond the reach of enemy anti-aircraft fire. Like an eggshell, the porcelain bomb would shatter into millions of tiny fragments, leaving no trace.[27] Although plague remained Ishii's agent of choice, Unit 731 also conducted research into the use of anthrax. The *Ha* bomb was designed to spread *B. anthracis* spores. It featured a thin steel wall and contained 1,500 cylindrical shot immersed in half-a-litre of anthrax mixture. The bomb's anti-personnel shrapnel effect on impact would create anthrax-infected wounds over a diameter of around 40 metres. Whereas the *Uji* was designed for use against civilians, the *Ha* was designed for battlefield use against troops.[28]

The Japanese Army authorized the first wartime BW attack when Japan was fighting the Soviet Union in a border war over Manchuria. On 12 July 1939, Ishii sent a special team into enemy territory to dump prepared salmonella and typhoid bacteria into the Halha River. The effectiveness of this operation was never determined.[29] A similar exercise, however, backfired badly when a release of cholera bacteria into a river resulted in the infection of Japanese troops, causing 10,000 casualties and 1,700 deaths.[30] On the whole, most Japanese biological attacks were unsuccessful. Nevertheless, by the end of the Second World War, Japanese germ warfare in more than 20 Chinese cities and provinces is estimated to have killed somewhere between 20,000 and 580,000 people.[31]

After its surrender in 1945, Japan levelled the BW experimentation areas, tried to destroy all documents concerning Unit 731, and swore participating scientists and officers to secrecy about its activities. In 1947, the US government secretly granted immunity from war crimes prosecution to Ishii and other participants in the Japanese BW programme. This was in exchange for exclusive acquisition of the programme's scientific data, especially the results of deadly experiments on human subjects. Senior Japanese officers provided information about their work on such diseases as botulism, influenza, plague, smallpox, tetanus, tularaemia, anthrax, cholera, TB and typhus.[32] Although the Soviet Union also used captured Japanese documents to improve its own BW programme,[33] it did prosecute Unit 731 personnel for war crimes. By contrast, in US-occupied post-war Japan, many former Unit 731 doctors and scientists went on to hold prominent positions at Japanese pharmaceutical and chemical companies. In August 2005, the *Japan Times* reported that, in addition to granting Unit 731 staff immunity from war crimes prosecution, the US government provided them with money, gifts, entertainment and other kinds of rewards. The total amount paid was equivalent to between 20 million and 40 million yen today.[34]

The secret deal for the US to acquire the BW technology employed by Japan during its occupation of China was exposed in 1980 by American journalist John Powell, who had obtained memoranda exchanged between US General Douglas MacArthur and his staff.[35] Two years later, Japan officially acknowledged its wartime BW programme and the fact that Ishii had received a large retirement pension.[36] To this day, however, Japanese archives concerning Unit 731 remain closed to independent researchers. The significance of the US decision to acquire Japanese BW data is uncertain. One view is that information from Japanese experiments obtained after 1945 would have done little to enhance American knowledge of BW. The United States had established its own BW programme in 1943 which, within a year, had arguably exceeded the expertise of Unit 731.[37] Perhaps granting immunity to Unit 731 personnel was simply a means of keeping their BW knowledge from the Soviet Union. On the other hand, the Japanese data would have been extremely valuable, particularly as it was the first ever to describe the results of experiments with pathogenic agents on human subjects.[38]

According to Ken Alibek, a defector from the former Soviet Union's BW programme, information on the Unit 731 programme 'convinced Washington that biological weapons could be developed in greater quantities and with far greater effectiveness than anyone had suspected'.[39] A confidential memorandum, dated 1 July 1947, circulated to US military and State Department officials, contained the statement: 'The value to US of Japanese BW data is of such importance to national security as to far outweigh the value accruing from war crimes prosecution.'[40] Whatever Washington's motivations were at the time for acquiring Japanese knowledge of BW, this decision would come back to haunt the United States when it was accused a few years later of deploying BW during the Korean War.

Korean War allegations

In February 1952, North Korean foreign minister Bak Hun Yung and Chinese Premier Zhou Enlai attracted worldwide attention when they made the allegation that the United States deployed BW on an experimental basis in China and North Korea during the Korean War. At the time, Western governments dismissed it as hostile propaganda based largely on forced confessions from captured US Air Force pilots.[41] In their book, *The United States and Biological Warfare*, authors Stephen Endicott and Edward Hagerman draw on declassified American, British and Canadian documents to argue that the United States employed an operational BW system in the Korean War. The authors place this documentary evidence alongside information drawn from the medical and operational archives of the Chinese and North Korean armies in the field. They observe a pattern of disease and delivery systems consistent with American BW capabilities, but anomalous with local incidence of naturally occurring disease. The evidence cited is corroborative and circumstantial rather than direct, and the authors' arguments feature a certain amount of conjecture. For example, in asking why the Chinese and North Koreans did not use the archival material to reinforce their accusation in 1952, the authors speculate that the two countries did not wish to expose intelligence information that the United States might have used to assess the effectiveness of their BW experiments.[42] The reasoning behind such speculation is somewhat circular in the way it assumes the very point at issue: that BW experiments were in fact going on.

Endicott and Hagerman point to the belief of the US military that a great advantage of biological warfare would be the enemy's difficulty in distinguishing it from naturally occurring diseases, especially given the poor sanitary conditions of the enemy's territory.[43] This very factor, however, could be used to support an argument that deliberate disease never occurred in China and North Korea. Rather, outbreaks of diseases endemic to the area were probably natural occurrences resulting from the disruption of war, crowding, an increase in the mobility of the population, a breakdown of sanitation, and a lack of pest control and adequate medical services.[44] Endicott and Hagerman also describe five isolated cases of inhalation anthrax, without occupational exposure, occurring in China during the war.[45] Today, the absence of occupational exposure in even a single case of inhalation anthrax would cause alarm regarding possible BW use. However, cases of non-occupational inhalation anthrax can occur. And if *B. anthracis* spores really were deliberately spread by US forces, it is difficult to believe that such exercises would have killed only one person at each targeted site.[46]

Based on American documents, some of the circumstantial evidence to suggest the United States used BW during the Korean War is that:

1   the US Army's Special Operations Division at Fort Detrick at the time produced biological agents and delivery systems;
2   the US Air Force headquarters had a special division that, among other things, directed and supervised covert BW operations; and
3   that it had a specially trained air wing sent to the Far East to carry out its tasks.

From the other side, Endicott and Hagerman cite evidence in Chinese archives that:

1   the United States produced disease-bearing insects, and disease-bearing insects were discovered in Northeast Asia;
2   it prepared infected bird feathers, and feathers appeared in China near exploded bombs; and
3   there was an overlap in the diseases cultivated by the United States and those diagnosed in China and North Korea.[47]

Putting this evidence together, Endicott and Hagerman contend that the US programme of BW experiments was 'too large and too complex an operation, and was possessed of too much inner logic, to have been concocted by the Communist side for propaganda purposes, as some have suggested'.[48] It is true that the Chinese did obtain confessions from 25 captured US pilots saying that they had participated in biological warfare experiments. However, interspersed with the technical detail about BW delivery methods was a good deal of communist rhetoric. This led most observers to doubt that the confessions had been written by those supposedly testifying to them. All the confessions were renounced when the pilots returned to the United States after the war.[49]

The allegation that the United States deployed BW during the Korean War was most probably an exercise in propaganda of huge and elaborate proportions. In January 1998, a reporter for the Japanese newspaper *Sankei Shimbun* published the findings of 12 documents from former Soviet archives that provide detailed evidence that the allegations were contrived.[50] Unfortunately, the documents had to be copied by hand in the Russian Presidential Archive, then translated. As a result, without the signs of authenticity that photocopies provide – such as seals, stamps or signatures – the accuracy of the documents will inevitably be questioned until the originals are formally released. In any event, the documents describe remarkable measures taken by the North Koreans and Chinese, with Soviet advice, to create false evidence to corroborate their charges against the United States. Moreover, publicly available documents from the Russian Foreign Ministry Archive indicate that Soviet officials were involved in managing the North Korean propaganda campaign about US use of BW so as to prevent the falsity of the claims from being revealed.[51]

The work of Endicott and Hagerman, while presenting evidence highly suggestive of BW use, is ultimately unsatisfying on the vital question of whether the United States in fact used BW in the Korean War. The United States had the means and the opportunity to deploy BW, but only the release of engagement reports (if they exist at all) might finally settle this issue. Similarly, more documentation regarding the veracity of the original allegations against the United States, particularly from China, is needed to give a full account of whether and to what extent this was a massive propaganda campaign.

Myanmar allegations

In addition to the Korean War allegations, accusations that the Myanmar military used BW against minority peoples in the early 1990s are also problematic. The allegation is generally absent from the literature on BW, although Myanmar country-specialist Andrew Selth discusses it in a 1999 publication.[52] The purpose of including the Myanmar allegations in this chapter is simply to illustrate further the difficulties of proving that BW have been used.

One piece of circumstantial evidence is that, between 1978 and 1989, 15 Myanmar army officers received training in protection against nuclear, biological and chemical warfare at a military academy in West Germany.[53] From this it could be inferred that Myanmar had sought to acquire the capability to protect its own troops while deploying BW in a battlefield setting. However, a more innocent and likely explanation would be that Myanmar was seeking the capability to protect its military personnel against biological attacks by an enemy state. Other evidence is reported, dating from 1993, of strange white boxes with parachutes being dropped near villages, and people in the drop area becoming sick up to two weeks later with a disease resembling cholera or shigella. In late 1994, an investigating team from the human rights group Christian Solidarity International suggested that the white boxes contained disease-causing bacteria and were intended for release over villages sympathetic to insurgent groups in eastern Myanmar. However, when sample white boxes were examined by independent scientists in Thailand and Canada, they were found to be harmless pressure-measuring devices routinely used in meteorological work. An alternative explanation for the mysterious disease outbreaks in eastern Myanmar in 1993 is that, as neighbouring Thailand and Bangladesh had experienced a particularly virulent strain of cholera around that time, the disease had simply spread to Myanmar naturally.[54]

The claim that Myanmar has used BW sits uneasily with the reality that the country has very few facilities for research into infectious diseases. It is also doubtful whether the Myanmar leadership would have deployed a BW agent which, if contagious, could have overwhelmed the country's frail health system and spread across the border to Thailand, potentially bringing grave political consequences. On balance, the circumstantial evidence of BW use by Myanmar in the past is unconvincing, and the existence of a BW programme today is highly unlikely. Other countries in East Asia are more capable than Myanmar of running a BW programme, although capability is distinct from intention. The next section explores this notion by assessing whether it is appropriate to regard present-day North Korea and China as BW states.

North Korea and China: the 'usual suspects'

Any assessment of a country's BW status must be preceded by two important caveats. First, compared to conventional and nuclear capabilities, there is little information publicly available on state-based BW programmes. This is unsurprising as BW are banned under international law. Second, information in the English language tends to be dominated by US intelligence assessments, the accuracy of which is open to question – after its invasion of Iraq in 2003, it emerged that the United States had failed to assess accurately the nature and scope of the pre-war Iraqi BW programme. This is not to suggest, however, that non-US assessments would necessarily be more accurate. Rather, establishing a state's BW status is inherently difficult in general. To 'possess' BW means more than simply having the means of producing biological agents. A militarily significant BW capability would also require, among other things, tried and tested systems for disseminating agents, plans and procedures for BW operations, and an established network of logistical support. These elements are what would crucially indicate offensive intent in addition to mere capability. In the case of North Korea and China, the 'usual suspects' in East Asia, intent is virtually impossible to determine reliably.

North Korea

What little information there is about North Korean BW has come from defectors. Although such sources are uncertain, North Korea's closed system of government means there is little reliable information to be derived from other sources. Defectors have differed in their accounts of the extent of BW weaponization, but it is generally believed that North Korea has been pursuing a BW capability since the 1960s and has had an offensive arsenal of some kind since the 1970s. Sources from the US, Russian and South Korean governments agree that North Korea has a BW programme, although there is no consensus on whether it has gone beyond research and development to the production of actual weapons.[55] US and Russian official assessments are characterized by cautious language and a lack of hard information. For example, a recent US Central Intelligence Agency (CIA) report assessed that North Korea possesses equipment, supplies and agents that 'could be used' to support a BW programme, its munitions production infrastructure 'would have allowed' North Korea to weaponize BW agents and the country 'may have' such weapons available for use.[56] Other US government reports note that North Korea is capable of producing agents like anthrax, plague, cholera and smallpox, but they do not specify the size of a North Korean BW stockpile or the existence of BW facilities. A Russian intelligence report that North Korea is researching these agents left open the possibility that such work is for defensive purposes.[57]

Assessments derived from South Korean sources tend to be more expansive. In December 2001, the South Korean Ministry of National Defense produced a map showing the locations of suspected BW facilities in North Korea – three for BW production and six for research. However, very little is known about these facilities, such as precisely which micro-organisms are being researched, produced and weaponized, if at all.[58] With regard to information from non-government sources, Elisa Harris has observed that some claims about the size and scope of North Korea's BW programme are manifestly unreliable.[59] For example, a 2002 article in the *Korean Journal of Defense Analysis* stated that North Korea's BW inventory comprised at least ten agents (cholera, pest, anthrax, typhoid, diphtheria, typhus, haemorrhagic fever, botulism, yellow fever and brucellosis), but it did not cite a source for this information.[60] On the issue of BW delivery, South Korean sources estimate that 30 per cent of North Korea's artillery pieces are capable of firing BW warheads.[61] This sits uneasily with US technical assessments that live biological agents degrade significantly when placed in the high acceleration environment of an artillery shell.[62] However, North Korea might have more efficient means of delivering BW. Joseph Bermudez argues that North Korea's numerous An-2 COLT aircraft would be an excellent delivery system for BW due to their slow speed, ability to fly low and largely undetected, and load-carrying capabilities.[63] North Korea also possesses several types of short-range land-, air- and sea-launched anti-ship cruise missiles which are potential means of BW delivery.[64] One recent assessment is that both North Korea and China possess the capability to convert the anti-ship HY-4 cruise missile into a 500 or 1,000 kilometre-range weapon carrying a BW payload of 300 kg or 120 kg respectively.[65] Nevertheless, there appears to be no evidence on the public record to indicate that either country has succeeded in marrying missile technology with the technical requirements for efficient biological agent dispersal.

In assessing North Korea's BW status, as is the case with Myanmar, an important final consideration is that such weapons are potentially a greater threat to North Korea than to its enemies because of the country's limited medical capabilities. North Korea is ill-equipped to deal with an in-kind retaliation or a BW rebound that might occur, for example, if a highly contagious agent were deliberately spread in a nearby country. Its healthcare resources are already under great strain without the additional burden of infectious disease, and local capacity to produce pharmaceuticals is very limited.[66]

China (and Taiwan)

When China became a member of the BWC in 1984 it declared that, having once been the victim of BW, it had not produced or possessed such weapons and would never do so in the future. US intelligence sources believe, however, that China started an offensive BW programme in the 1950s and has likely retained elements of that programme. Using cautious language, a January 2001 US government report assessed that China possessed a sufficiently advanced biotechnology infrastructure to 'allow' it to develop and produce biological agents, and a munitions industry sufficient to 'allow' it to use a variety of means that 'could be used' for BW delivery. The report also noted that 'China's declarations under the voluntary BWC declarations for confidence building purposes are believed to be inaccurate and incomplete'.[67] On this point, however, the United States itself was caught out eight months later – in September 2001, the *New York Times* revealed that the US government had failed to declare three projects of dubious BWC legality.[68] These are discussed in detail in Chapter 9.

In a more recent unclassified report to the US Congress, the CIA expressed concern over China acting as a supplier of nuclear, missile, chemical and conventional weapon technology and materials, but the report made no mention of China being a supplier of BW.[69] Like North Korea, China produces several types of land-, sea- and air-launched cruise missiles, which are potential means of BW delivery. Most are short-range anti-ship missiles, although China is also developing land-attack cruise missiles and a submarine-launched anti-ship cruise missile.[70] According to US military technology assessments, however, certain Chinese cruise missile models are unlikely candidates for conversion to BW delivery. The Silkworm, for example, leaves a turbulent airflow in its wake, which makes it difficult to deliver a sprayed pathogen.[71]

If indeed China is investigating offensive applications of biological agents, one possible motivation is that it believes neighbouring Taiwan has developed BW of its own. According to Russian intelligence, Taiwan is possibly conducting a BW research programme, and the Canadian Security and Intelligence Service believes Taiwan has developed three dozen types of bacteria, apparently for weaponization purposes.[72] If so, China might feel it needs a defensive capability as well as the means to retaliate in kind to a Taiwanese BW attack. As Taiwan is unable to obtain member status under the BWC, it is not bound by the Convention's provisions and does not have the opportunity to participate officially in confidence-building measures such as declarations of potentially BW-relevant facilities. During the 2003 SARS outbreak, it was revealed that Taiwan had a secret biological warfare research centre, the military-run Institute of Preventive Medical Research (IPMR). Taiwanese President Chen Shui-Bian made the revelation to media while announcing that he had ordered the IPMR to work on a cure for SARS. The facility is reportedly capable of producing weapons-grade biological agents, although Taiwanese officials claim it exists only to research ways of preventing biological attacks from mainland China.[73] Beyond producing biological agents, however, it could be difficult for Taiwan to develop a fully-operational BW programme. Given the small size of this densely populated island, it is unlikely that Taiwan's military has been able to train in the use of such weapons or to test their effectiveness safely.[74]

Conclusion

There is an overarching theme regarding the science and history of deliberate disease. Whether one is contemplating the effects of a biological attack, the true military value of BW, allegations of BW use, or whether a country possesses BW, each issue is characterized by profound uncertainty. What is clear, however, is that it is inappropriate to regard BW simply as 'weapons of mass destruction'. For reasons related to biological agent choice and circumstances of delivery, BW effects are diverse in nature and scale. And using deliberate disease to achieve mass casualties would be far less straightforward than using the only true WMD – nuclear weapons. The science and technology underlying BW, the diversity of biological agents and their effects, and the challenges of delivering them efficiently are factors relevant to their military value. On the whole, BW have little tactical utility, although in some circumstances they could generate psychological casualties or disrupt enemy operations. At the strategic level, BW are no substitute for a nuclear capability. For the purposes of deterrence in particular, the value of BW is undermined by two fundamental uncertainties – whether a country in fact possesses BW, and whether a biological attack would inflict unacceptable damage.

The story of BW in East Asia includes instances and allegations of BW use in the past, and possible possession in the present. The campaign of biological warfare waged by Imperial Japan before and during the Second World War was the largest of its kind in history. However, this might also have been the last time BW were in fact used in the region – allegations of BW use during the Korean War and in Myanmar have not been proven. These allegations do, however, illustrate the difficulty of distinguishing between deliberate and natural disease outbreaks. It is difficult also to determine whether a given country today possesses BW. North Korea and China are routinely cited as BW suspects in East Asia; however, there is little hard evidence to support this. Defectors have described in some detail North Korea's past BW activities, so it is reasonable to suspect Pyongyang might retain some relevant materials and equipment to this day. However, whether North Korea would ever want or need to use BW is doubtful. The country's health system is ill-equipped to cope if a biological attack went wrong or if an adversary decided to retaliate in kind, and the Pyongyang regime might regard its conventional and nuclear capabilities as sufficient to ensure its survival. With regard to China, the case is even weaker. There is little evidence regarding the existence and nature of an offensive Chinese BW programme in the past, and in fact China expressly repudiated this notion when it joined the BWC. Published US intelligence assessments emphasize China's capability to produce and use BW, but they present no evidence to indicate that this is wedded to hostile intent.

Any state that did match requisite technical capability with hostile intent to use BW would be a serious security threat. A less certain threat, to be explored in the next chapter, is that of biological attacks perpetrated by non-state actors.

6 Biological attacks and the non-state perpetrator[1]

Assessing the willingness and ability of non-state actors to use BW is difficult, largely because there have been very few confirmed cases of groups or individuals acquiring or employing biological agents. Faced with the uncertainty associated with a paucity of empirical data on non-state use of BW, many policy-makers tend to err on the side of regarding the threat potential as high. They seek to hedge against the possibility of someone exploiting the full catastrophic potential of BW. In particular, policy discussions of 'terrorism' are often characterized by a pessimistic outlook formed by a belief that nightmarish hypothetical scenarios will become a reality. But assuming the worst, while analytically and politically convenient, is an expensive and possibly counterproductive way to approach the problem of biological attacks by non-state actors. In the interests of accurate threat assessment and appropriate resource allocation, it is incumbent on policy-makers and scholars alike to go beyond canvassing all the ghastly possibilities of 'bioterrorism'. Stepping away from strict pessimism, it is important to explore why particular individuals or groups would not and/or could not carry out a mass-casualty biological attack. This in turn facilitates greater appreciation of how to address the prospect of small-scale BW use – the most likely scenario when contemplating non-state perpetrators.

This chapter is presented in three sections. The first discusses some possible motivations for and disincentives against carrying out a biological attack. The second section explores the technical challenges likely to be encountered by a non-state actor that decides to embark on a BW venture. And the final section is a case study of the Japanese Aum Shinrikyo cult which, although motivated to conduct a well-resourced programme for deliberately causing disease, was incapable of achieving a single BW casualty.

Disease as a weapon of choice

For state and non-state actors alike, the technical challenges of biological agent production and efficient delivery, as well as the inevitable delayed effect of a BW attack, are relevant considerations as to whether deliberate disease is worth pursuing. However, would-be non-state perpetrators of biological attacks also face a different set of factors in deciding whether to select the BW option. These factors arise from the resource and organizational deficiencies of non-state entities as compared to states, the different modes by which they pursue interests and objectives, and from the fact that non-state actors are not bound by international law.

Motivating factors

For a non-state actor seeking to avoid capture or retaliation, the advantage of a biological attack is that it could be carried out covertly. A BW release via non-explosive means would almost certainly go unnoticed unless the attack was announced by its perpetrator. Thus suspicions of a BW attack would likely not be aroused until patients started presenting unusual disease symptoms at numerous clinics and hospitals in the target country. By that point, managing the effects of the attack could be extremely difficult, particularly if a contagious agent were used. Public health systems around the world are already stretched to the limit dealing with naturally occurring infectious diseases, as well as with non-infectious illnesses. Hospitals would have to deal with patients actually exposed to a BW agent as well as uninfected people demanding medical attention just in case. The phenomenon of the 'worried well' relates to the most attractive feature of BW as regards non-state motivations: the great human dread of infection would act as a multiplier in terms of the effects generated by even a small-scale biological attack.

People are acutely sensitive to the prospect of infection, as distinct from other health risks in everyday life such as smoking and high fat consumption. In addition, we tend to distinguish between *types* of infection based on the historical reputation of a disease, whether it is characterized by grotesque symptoms and/or high fatality rates, and how common or familiar it is. Cities function normally in the midst of a community-wide epidemic of regular influenza. But an outbreak of plague, responsible for the fourteenth-century Black Death in Europe, would likely cause widespread panic. And the highly lethal Ebola virus, although not easily transmitted between humans, inspires particular dread because it causes massive haemorrhaging in its victims. New or unfamiliar diseases can also engender a level of fear out of proportion to the threat they pose, in morbidity and mortality terms, relative to other diseases. This is demonstrated by the panic reactions of many in China to the 2003 SARS outbreak, which ultimately caused fewer than 400 Chinese deaths. People's ancient and visceral fear of infectious disease is compounded by the notion that someone would deliberately contaminate them and, if the biological agent is contagious, that they in turn might contaminate others.[2] Moreover, that fear could be magnified even further by uncertainty – unlike a conventional explosion where the casualty count is immediately apparent, it is unlikely that anyone would immediately know the source and nature of a BW attack or the number of victims.

Some non-state actors might be particularly attracted to BW, over other forms of weaponry, because of the prominence of disease in some religious texts. In AD 570 (the birth year of Mohammed, the Prophet of Islam), an Abyssinian army attacked Mecca for the purpose of destroying the Kaaba, a shrine sacred to Arabs. According to the Koran, God sent flocks of birds that showered the Abyssinians with stones, producing sores that spread like a pestilence.[3] In the Bible's Book of Exodus the fifth plague used by God to punish Pharaoh was *murrain*, a group of cattle diseases that includes anthrax.[4] And in the 'Book of Revelations', 'Pestilence' is numbered as one of the Four Horsemen of the Apocalypse. Accordingly, a group might set out to use disease deliberately in order to mimic and please God. A number of authors identify extremist religious groups, especially those with apocalyptic visions, as the most likely perpetrators of biological attacks. Such groups may display an attitude to violence and mass death that bypasses normal societal sensibilities. They may be less likely to feel constrained by fear of a public backlash, since their actions are intended to please a Supreme Being and themselves, not to impress a secular constituency. And their victims, being outside their religious worldview, may be viewed as subhuman.[5] In the case of the Japanese cult Aum Shinrikyo, apocalyptic visions were a likely factor behind its efforts to produce and disseminate BW in the early 1990s. The cult's motivation to use BW is examined further in the final section of this chapter.

A scan of recorded BW events involving non-state actors suggests, however, that even a strongly religious element within an organization does not necessarily mean it will pursue some kind of disease-driven apocalypse. To the extent that religiously motivated organizations also have a political goal – for example, the establishment of an Islamic state – they are likely to encounter more earthly constraints. When US-based members of the Rajneesh cult contaminated restaurant salad bars with salmonella bacteria in 1984, they were pursuing a tangible political end rather than an apocalyptic goal. Their actions caused 751 cases of diarrhoeal illness, but resulted in no deaths. Concerned about land-use regulations in Wasco County, Oregon, the cult wanted to affect the outcome of elections for county commissioners in a way that would be favourable to the cult's plans to construct a new international headquarters.[6] In general, politico-religious groups would need to factor in popular reactions to their violence and the form it takes. This does not exclude the possibility of a biological attack, although it provides such groups with a reason to refrain from such action.

Moving beyond tentative judgements based on scarce empirical evidence, a model formulated by Daniel Gressang is a useful conceptual starting point for identifying the kind of non-state actors likely to be interested in BW. In assessing potential non-state use of 'WMD', Gressang adopts the fundamental tenet that all 'terrorists' alike seek to acquire and maintain some degree of influence over an identifiable audience, broadly defined. For example, Osama bin Laden might make pronouncements about the need to liberate holy Muslim lands from infidel occupation. In so doing, his intended audience at one level might be God, but bin Laden may also be reaching out to at least three earthly audiences: the US government, the American people and the global Islamic community.[7] The WMD potential of a non-state group, Gressang argues, is determined by a communicative dynamic between it and its audience which turns on three factors:

1   the type of audience, human or ethereal, to which the group is appealing;
2   the content of the group's message (whether it calls for destruction rather than change); and
3   the degree of social interaction the group engages in.

According to Gressang's model, WMD potential is greatest where the group:

1   is appealing to an ethereal audience (a Supreme Being);
2   has a message of destruction (for example, of a state or race); and
3   has an inapposite, minimalist relationship with the rest of society.[8]

Gressang's model is useful when contemplating the motivation of non-state actors to cause mass casualties, although it lacks two important contextual elements. First, in using the cover-all term 'WMD', the model does not provide scope for considering why a group or individual might prefer to use BW rather than nuclear or chemical weapons. In addition to the sheer number of casualties to be achieved, the *type* of casualties caused might also be relevant to an attacker's motivations. As discussed above, disease-based casualties might hold a particular fascination for some religiously motivated organizations. Also, the focus on 'mass destruction' excludes the possibility of small-scale BW attacks which, for reasons to be discussed later in this chapter, are a more likely scenario. Second, there is arguably a close relationship between the motivation to use certain weapons and the technical ability to do so. Thus, Gressang's model could be improved by adding a fourth dimension: capability. With regard to BW, it is conceivable that a group would regard the complexities of production and delivery as a major disincentive.

Disincentives

Although deliberate disease may be regarded as a powerful generator of dread, there are also reasons why many existing non-state groups might rule out the use of BW. For those pursuing clear political aims in a given territorial area, such an attack would not generally appeal. This is because the group's own constituency could be put at risk, especially if a highly contagious agent were deployed. For example, a BW attack in Ireland would affect Catholics as well as Protestants, and an attack in Israel would affect Arabs as well as Jews. Long-standing and conspicuous non-state organizations such as the Irish Republican Army and Hamas, rather than being bent on perpetrating maximum harm at every turn, are restrained by political vision, operational practices and moral codes from seeking and using unconventional weapons. In some cases, group leaders have specifically indicated to their members that the use of biological or chemical weapons would not be legitimate to their struggle.[9]

Other disincentives against non-state actors using BW, a widely loathed form of weaponry, include the risks of provoking a massive government crackdown and alienating present and potential supporters – although this would of course depend upon BW use being accurately attributed to the perpetrator. At a more practical level, biological agents are inherently dangerous to use without special equipment and their effects are difficult to control after deployment. Agent preparation and efficient delivery can present enormous technical challenges, and non-state actors with limited resources may well be averse to failure. These considerations might lead a group to conclude that it is better to repeat methods that have proven successful in the past, and that are more reliable than BW. This would see conventional bombs, which provide instant explosive gratification, remain the non-state aggressor's weapons of choice.

If a non-state organization's purpose is simply to convey a message to its human audience, mass casualties might not be necessary. Rather, it would be enough to carry out a conspicuous attack that produced a great deal of noise and/or disruption. By contrast, a biological attack would, by its very nature, be silent. And, as the disease caused by a biological agent would take time to incubate inside victims' bodies and possibly spread to others, the effects would be delayed and gradual. This means an attack of this kind (assuming it could be distinguished from a naturally occurring infectious disease outbreak) would lack a single catastrophic moment for the news media to focus upon along with the political message, if any, to be conveyed by the perpetrator. Indeed, were a contagious biological agent deployed, journalists and camera crews might not even be able to access a BW-affected area because of quarantine and isolation restrictions. On the other hand, the silence and delayed effect of a biological attack could be attractive for a non-state group wishing to avoid detection. And 'theatrical' considerations might matter little to groups with an apocalyptic bent for whom mass casualties, achieved by whatever means, are the true objective – announcing that a BW attack has occurred would be dramatic, but it would also alert the intended victims and stimulate medical interventions to mitigate the extent of human damage.

Carrying out a biological attack

Once a non-state organization has decided, for whatever reason, that engaging in deliberate disease is a good way to achieve its aims, there remains the issue of having the capability to carry out a biological attack successfully. In the literature on BW, there is no shortage of descriptions of non-state actors possessing nightmarish capabilities. For example, in their book *Living Terrors,* Michael Osterholm and John Schwarz present attack scenarios including:

- a disgruntled laboratory worker who grows anthrax bacteria in an abandoned farmhouse then disperses it in a crop duster over a sport stadium;
- a hospital worker who steals a deadly strain of *E. coli* bacteria and uses it to poison the food of hundreds of schoolchildren; and
- a former Soviet scientist who grows smallpox virus in fertilized chicken eggs, sprays it through a shopping mall air-conditioning system, then watches the disease spread through the United States.[10]

However, less attention has been devoted to assessing dispassionately whether hypothetical scenarios are likely to be transformed into reality. 'Dark Winter', an exercise conducted in the United States in June 2001, presented participants with a hypothetical scenario of three smallpox-laden aerosol clouds infecting 1,000 people each in shopping malls in Oklahoma City, Atlanta and Philadelphia.[11] The scenario controversially assumed that a non-state perpetrator could actually obtain smallpox, samples of which are extremely rare, and then spread enough particles efficiently to infect 3,000 people. In an exercise along similar lines, a group of senior European and American politicians gathered in Washington, DC in January 2005 to participate in 'Atlantic Storm'. The scenario included a fictional group called Al Jihad Al Jadid releasing smallpox (sourced from a microbiology facility in the former Soviet Union) at major transport hubs around the world, causing the infection of 84,000 people.[12] Some scientists complained afterwards that 'Atlantic Storm' was based on unrealistic assumptions, especially as regards the capability of 'terrorists' to acquire, mass-produce and disseminate the smallpox virus.[13] Both 'Atlantic Storm' and 'Dark Winter' served to focus attention on the prospect of mass casualties, whereas technical considerations and historical experience suggest that this is the least likely consequence of a non-state biological attack.

Opinion is divided as regards the ease and expense of acquiring a BW capability. Walter Laqueur has observed a belief among some authors that an undergraduate biology student could easily produce biological agents in a garage or kitchen, and that making BW is as easy as brewing beer – others believe a higher degree and greater variety of expertise is required, in areas including microbiology, aerosol physics, pathology and pharmacology, and that a BW project would require access to a sophisticated laboratory.[14] Ultimately, assessments of non-state BW capabilities depend largely upon the scale of biological attack being contemplated. Malcolm Dando's assessment is that 'all the evidence in the open literature strongly suggests that it is very difficult to achieve effective distribution of an agent in order to cause mass human casualties'.[15] However, for threat-assessment purposes, it would be a mistake to focus on the requirements for a state-run offensive BW programme designed to launch massive quantities of aerosolized biological agents, and then to simply dismiss inferior non-state capabilities. In the realm of biological attacks and the non-state perpetrator, there is an important 'non-WMD' dimension.

Documented BW attacks by non-state perpetrators have been small in scale and have generally produced fewer casualties than conventional explosives. But success need not be measured in terms of casualties alone. Because the notion of deliberate infection generates such immense fear in people, a non-state perpetrator can potentially achieve large-scale disruption and consternation even with a crudely delivered biological agent that affects only a few victims directly. Richard Danzig argues that, short of 'catastrophic bioterrorism', a campaign of small-scale attacks could severely tax the target society: 'Biological terrorism affords the possibility of repeated attack, undermining confidence and forcing ever-escalating investments of resources to achieve a modicum of defense.'[16] The significance of successive, small-scale biological attacks is illustrated by the October 2001 anthrax envelope attacks that killed five people and infected 17 others in the United States. An important feature of these attacks was that the letters laced with *B. anthracis* bacteria instructed the reader to take antibiotics. Arguably, by announcing that a biological attack was underway, the perpetrator intended that direct human damage would be limited. Nevertheless, as a result of the attacks, antibiotics were prescribed to thousands of people, and rumours and copycat hoaxes occupied emergency and law-enforcement services throughout the world.

To assess further the challenges a non-state actor faces in seeking to carry out a biological attack, the remainder of this section examines:

1   the prospect of sponsorship (intended or inadvertent) by states;
2   the technical hurdles for would-be non-state perpetrators seeking to cause deliberate disease without state assistance; and
3   a brief case study of the extent to which Muslim militants in Southeast Asia pose a BW threat.

State sponsorship

At various times throughout history, states have sought to further their national interests by sponsoring violent acts by non-state entities. The tools for this violence have generally been restricted to conventional armaments. By contrast, for a state to place a BW capability in the hands of a group not entirely within that state's control would generally be too great a risk, especially if the particular biological agent and its delivery system could generate mass casualties. To the contrary, Avigdor Haselkorn has argued that there is only a slight degree of difference between providing BW to a specific non-state organization and a state leader delegating launch authority to military commanders; both are a risk to the regime. Saddam Hussein's 1990 delegation decision, for example, might indicate that the Iraqi president would not have been averse to handing BW to a non-state group if faced with an unwinnable confrontation.[17] For most other authors, however, the notion of a state sponsoring non-state BW use is highly problematic.[18] Bearing in mind that only groups of an extreme and possibly apocalyptic nature are likely to employ BW, a state might fear loss of control or treachery – could a BW-capable group be entirely trusted not to cause disease in the sponsor state's own territory? Moreover, the discovery of links between a BW incident and a state sponsor might also attract disastrous retaliation by the target country. Whether for fear of disloyalty, incompetence or indiscretion, any state anxious for its own survival would be unlikely to entrust a BW capability to ruthless outsiders.

On the other hand, it is conceivable that a state could be the unwitting sponsor of a non-state biological attack. The October 2001 attacks in the United States reportedly featured *B. anthracis* in high-grade powder form – the several grams inside envelopes sent to US Senators Tom Daschle and Patrick Leahy were prepared so that most of the particles were under 5 microns in diameter and treated to facilitate aerosolization.[19] Moreover, the anthrax spores contained in all the attacker's envelopes were known variants of the Ames strain, which first became available to the US biodefence establishment in the early 1980s.[20] This evidence raises the possibility that one or more military insiders used their position to steal bacterial samples and attack the United States with its own anthrax.

Crop dusters and 'suicide sneezers'

For would-be non-state perpetrators without access to state resources, a biological attack must be prepared from scratch. In 1999–2000, the US Defense Threat Reduction Agency demonstrated that a small facility for producing biological agents could be built using commercially available materials at a cost of US$1.6 million.[21] To cause mass casualties, however, it is not enough simply to be able to grow a biological agent. In addition, the agent must be kept alive, it must be of a strain that is lethal to humans, it must be disseminated in an aerosol form consisting of particles of a size suitable for inhalation, and the attack perpetrator must have some understanding of the meteorological conditions at the target. Two oft-cited means by which an individual or group might cause deliberate disease are biological agent dissemination using crop-spraying aircraft and the deployment of so-called 'suicide sneezers'.

A CIA report published in 2003 expressed concern that 'al-Qa'ida has explored the possibility of using agricultural aircraft for large-area dissemination of biological warfare agents such as anthrax'.[22] Although the requirement of precise particle sizes (1–5 microns) to infect human lungs means that this scenario of non-state BW delivery is generally unrealistic, there is evidence to suggest the threat cannot be dismissed altogether. Aerial crop spraying is carried out under specific conditions in order to avoid off-target delivery of pesticides. These include using large droplets (about 150 microns in diameter), minimizing agent release height and spraying with a crosswind greater than 7.2 km/h but less than 15 km/h. Thermal or inversion weather conditions can result in significant off-target droplet movement, and high-speed winds have the potential to increase the distance droplets travel downwind.[23] All these factors, and large droplet size in particular, militate against efficient BW delivery. On the other hand, biological agent dissemination using an agricultural sprayer may still produce a small number of particles within the size range suitable for inhalation. A 2003 article in *Biosecurity and Bioterrorism* summarized empirical data from Canada on human exposure that followed outdoor spraying of the insecticide agent *Bacillus thuringiensis*, a bacterium closely related to *B. anthracis*. Regarding the BW threat posed by crop-duster delivery, the study found that most of the aerosol would be dispensed in the agriculturally useful size range of 100–150 microns, but '[d]roplets of 2 to 7 microns are formed in sufficient quantities to penetrate houses and contaminate the nasal passages of residents inside their homes'.[24] Nevertheless, the quantity of respirable particles might be insufficient to cause illness and/or death – the estimated dose required to kill 50 per cent of exposed humans is between 2,500 and 55,000 anthrax spores.[25]

In 2002 the BBC screened a docu-drama, *Smallpox 2002: Silent Weapon*, in which a 'suicide patient' walking around New York City triggers a worldwide pandemic that leaves 60 million people dead.[26] Fortunately, initiating an epidemic by dispatching one or more infected hosts to a target population is not as straightforward as it sounds. The hosts might be too ill to withstand travel, or they might be recognized as having unfamiliar symptoms on or after arrival at their destination, thus triggering the suspicions of the target country. And even if a population were susceptible to a given disease, a few isolated cases might not be enough to guarantee an epidemic. In a naturally occurring disease outbreak, many infected people are epidemiological dead ends; that is, they or the people they contact fail to pass on the disease. To be effective, the deliberate causing of an epidemic might require repeated introductions of a contagious disease, but this would increase the probability of 'suicide sneezers' being detected.[27] It is still possible, however, that a biological attack could successfully be carried out in this way, especially if the target country were not generally vigilant regarding public health.

In any event, the human vector scenario depends heavily on the disease host consciously avoiding medical treatment for as long as possible so as to delay alerting public health authorities and to maximize the chance of disease transmission. On this point, the choice of disease is highly relevant – for example, an influenza infection is transmissible in its pre-symptomatic stage, whereas smallpox is not generally contagious before symptoms appear. If members of a non-state group were deployed as the *unwitting* hosts of a contagious biological agent during the disease's incubation period, they would have no reason to refuse medical treatment once they became sick. By contrast, a witting and determined host would be more likely to avoid medical attention. However, such a volunteer would be extremely rare. Adam Dolnik defines a suicide attack as 'a premeditated act of ideologically or religiously motivated violence, in which the success of the operation is contingent on self-inflicted death by the perpetrator(s) during the attack'.[28] He argues that someone willing to be a suicide bomber would not necessarily be willing to be a suicide sneezer; the difference lies in the manner of dying. Suicide bombers of Islamic faith, for example, are traditionally motivated by the promise of a quick and honourable death. There are reports of bombers smiling with joy prior to detonating their explosives and (they believe) entering the gates of heaven. By contrast, someone infected with Ebola or smallpox would not likely be smiling during the days or weeks it would take to succumb to the disease. This option, according to Dolnik, would seem much less heroic than a suicide bombing and would carry the unattractive risk of a prolonged and undignified death.[29] And, because the disease might not prove fatal, or medical intervention might occur, there would be no guarantee of the person achieving martyrdom.

The propensity of Muslim militants towards suicide bombings does not translate directly into an uncritical preparedness to be an infectious disease martyr. Regarding biological attacks in general, however, the case of Muslim militants in East Asia provides some useful insights into the relationship between non-state actors and BW.

Muslim militants in East Asia

There is little evidence on the public record to support the view that BW use by non-state organizations is a likely threat in Southeast Asia. Reported 'terrorist' involvement with BW has tended to consist of false alarms, or else has indicated only low-level interest. For example, in October 2003 Philippines security forces recovered a 'bio-terror manual' in a raid on a Jemaah Islamiyah (JI) hideout in the southern city of Cotabato, along with traces of powder thought to be a 'tetanus virus-carrying chemical'.[30] The powder turned out to be residue of a powerful explosive rather than a biological agent. And, according to Philippines health experts, even if the substance had contained *Clostridium tetanus* (which is a bacterium, not a virus), such an agent would not have been effective for BW purposes.[31] In May 2004, police in the Philippines captured from six suspected Abu Sayyaf Group members 'readings on biological and chemical warfare', although these were of a kind available on the public record rather than confidential military documents.[32] Muslim militants in general are able to access 'training materials' via the Internet, although these are typically not of high quality. The *Mujahideen Poisons Handbook*, for example, purports to explain how to manufacture 'beta-luminium poison.' There is no such thing, but perhaps the author was referring to botulinum toxin. In any case, the handbook instructs the reader to leave a mixture of flour, meat, fresh horse manure and water in a jar for ten days. In all likelihood, the result would be a bad smell rather than a dangerous biological agent.[33]

The CIA recently assessed that Al Qaeda's BW programme, although primarily focused on achieving mass casualty anthrax attacks, would most likely involve the use of other biological agents in smaller-scale attacks.[34] There is little evidence, however, that the organization has acquired pathogenic agents and worked out how to weaponize them, and no evidence that it has succeeded in a biological attack. Nevertheless, by simply letting people know of its interest in BW, Al Qaeda has succeeded in generating fear through publicity. This has included reports that agents of Al Qaeda in Southeast Asia were planning to set up an anthrax programme in Indonesia.[35]

On this point, it is worth noting that the extent to which Al Qaeda has an influence in Southeast Asia is a contested issue. Analysts of 'international terrorism', most notably Rohan Gunaratna, generally argue that Al Qaeda has recruited political organizations in Southeast Asia to its global 'jihadist' cause. Analysts who are country specialists, such as Sidney Jones, tend to emphasize how local groups of Muslim militants are able to act independently of Al Qaeda in pursuit of their own agenda. This difference in perspective is demonstrated by the case of JI. An internationalist might emphasize networks of individuals and point to the efforts of a man known as 'Hambali', reputedly Al Qaeda's senior agent in Southeast Asia, to forge operational links with JI. A country specialist might instead point out that the historical record does not establish that JI is in step with Al Qaeda, but rather is the successor to Indonesia's Darul Islam movement of the 1940s and 1950s.[36] On balance, the internationalist approach gives inadequate attention to the historical, political and cultural context in which so-called 'terrorist' organizations emerge and operate. That local context is highly relevant to whether a group would contemplate acquiring and using BW inside a particular country. When JI members targeted Westerners using conventional bombs in Bali in October 2002, the effects were indiscriminate enough to harm Indonesians and Indonesian interests as well. Given the nature of BW, it is difficult to imagine why a militant Islamic organization would prefer such weapons over explosives. The use of a biological agent inside Southeast Asia would be even less discriminating than bombings and, if it stimulated widespread contagion, would have largely uncontrollable adverse effects on the huge Muslim population in the region.

Whereas Muslim militants in Southeast Asia would be concerned for their politico-religious constituency, isolated and paranoid religious cults might be less squeamish about deliberate disease. To bring together the notions of motivation and capability, the final section of this chapter provides a case study of the BW programme run by the Japanese cult Aum Shinrikyo.

The case of Aum Shinrikyo

Aum Shinrikyo is best known as being responsible for the attack on the Tokyo subway in March 1995 using sarin (a chemical nerve agent). During the early 1990s, Aum also made several attempts to cause casualties using two biological agents, *Clostridium botulinum* and *B. anthracis*. The cult failed in this objective despite being able to operate under near-ideal conditions – it possessed ample finances, scientific expertise and well-equipped laboratories, and its activities went virtually undetected and undisturbed by Japanese law-enforcement authorities.

Founded in 1984 by Chizuo Matsumoto (a former yoga instructor), Aum Shinrikyo used front companies, high-pressure fundraising, insurance fraud and other criminal activities to become an organization of 10,000–60,000 members, with assets valued at between US$300 million and US$1 billion.[37] Its ideology was derived from a variety of sources, including Buddhism, Christianity, Shamanism, Hinduism and New Age beliefs. In its early years, Aum appears to have had earthly, political objectives. Matsumoto (also known as Shoko Asahara) and more than 20 of his followers stood for election to the Japanese parliament in 1989. According to some analysts, it was possibly Aum's collective feeling of humiliation at not being elected that led the cult's leader subsequently to pursue novel forms of weaponry and the overthrow of the established order.[38] Aum became a millenarian cult seeking to hasten Armageddon by precipitating a US nuclear attack on Japan. And Matsumoto, who regarded Nostradamus as a prophet, claimed to have supernatural powers and saw himself as a messiah who would lead his followers to safety as the end of the world drew near.[39]

Aum had a charismatic leader asserting divine authority, an apocalyptic world view, a fascination with violence and a collective paranoia amongst its members. These characteristics were arguably what predisposed the cult towards attempting extraordinary acts of violence such as using BW. Aum's BW programme was probably the largest and costliest ever conducted by a non-state organization. However, a caveat on the discussion that follows is that the Japanese authorities have to date released only limited information on the cult's activities. What little exists on the public record has mostly been distilled from trial proceedings involving cult members following the 1995 sarin attack. The picture of Aum's BW efforts is necessarily incomplete, although it seems clear that the cult encountered enormous difficulties, mostly technical, in its attempts to perpetrate biological attacks. In April 1990, Aum members drove a car around the Japanese Diet in Tokyo with the exhaust pipe fitted out to disseminate what was supposed to be botulinum toxin derived from *C. botulinum* bacteria. In early June 1993 they tried a similar exercise, this time with the goal of disrupting the wedding of Japan's Crown Prince Naruhito. Later that month, Aum members attempted to disseminate what they believed to be virulent anthrax bacteria from the roof of an eight-storey building owned by the cult. Although police received over 200 complaints about foul-smelling white fumes coming from Aum's building, they reportedly did not investigate inside.[40] None of these attacks had the desired effect of killing large numbers of people; it appears, rather, that they resulted in no deaths at all.

Understanding exactly why Aum's BW ventures failed is difficult due to the scarcity of unclassified data, although William Rosenau has suggested three main reasons:

1   the cult's anthrax bacteria and botulinum toxin were not lethal;
2   Aum had difficulties preparing these agents for dissemination and dispersing them; and
3   the organizational nature of the cult itself imposed limitations on Aum's BW efforts.[41]

In trial proceedings following his arrest, Seiichi Endo, Aum's 'Minister for Health and Welfare', testified that the cult's BW delivery methods had proven ineffective, and that its chosen strains of biological agents were not sufficiently virulent.[42] To avoid the technical challenges of turning *B. anthracis* spores into powder using large, expensive centrifuge and drying machines, Aum probably tried to disseminate its bacteria in liquid slurry form. This must be continuously refrigerated until it is used. And unless the slurry is extremely pure, material is likely to settle at the bottom of its container and so clog the sprayer used for dissemination. There is some evidence to suggest that Aum encountered problems keeping their dispersal devices from clogging. Around the time of the rooftop attacks in 1993, there were reports of a jelly-like substance scattered in the street nearby. This may have been clumps of bacterial culture medium (perhaps a blood agar substance), which would be likely to clog a sprayer device. Even if Aum's *B. anthracis* had been dangerous – it was, in fact, an attenuated animal vaccine strain of the bacteria – it could have been rendered harmless by adverse weather conditions at the time the attacks took place. Many appear to have been staged in the daytime, during Tokyo's warm summer months, when strong sunlight and smog were likely to have been present. Such weather conditions would have potentially reduced biological agent effectiveness.[43]

Rosenau suggests that cult-like organizations, those that seem to have the greatest interest in perpetrating biological attacks to achieve mass casualties, may be the least suited to meet the complex requirements for a BW programme. The Aum example illustrates that a paranoid, fantasy-prone and sometimes violent atmosphere is not conducive to the sound scientific judgements needed to produce and weaponize biological agents. Aum's leaders reinforced the cult's doctrines among members through the use of physical isolation, beatings, torture and the administration of hallucinogenic drugs such as LSD.[44] As an organization, Aum was also fickle by nature and inclined to embark on numerous expensive, and sometimes bizarre, ventures rather than concentrate on perfecting a particular weapon. Its activities in pursuit of producing mass-casualty effects included an expedition to acquire the Ebola virus during an outbreak in Zaire in October 1992.[45] Aum also attempted to build a high-power laser weapon and sought a device for generating earthquakes.[46] It is conceivable that, working inside an organization such as this, Aum's scientists simply had insufficient opportunity to develop and test a viable BW programme.

A final point to emphasize is that, when Aum conducted its biological attacks in the early 1990s, the Japanese authorities knew about the cult but were unwilling or unable to act. Aum's interest in deliberate disease was no secret – in early 1994, on a radio programme it sponsored in Russia, the cult had broadcast statements extolling the virtues of BW.[47] The ease with which Aum avoided the attention of the Japanese authorities is related to the cult's official religious status under Japan's Religious Corporation Law (1951). The Law grants official religions tax exemptions and a high degree of freedom from state intrusion. This special status partly explains the lax approach of the Japanese police towards Aum, even in the face of numerous complaints about suspicious activities.

Being left alone by the authorities and possessing ample financial resources could be considered near-ideal conditions for engaging in a BW project. Thus Aum's failure to cause a single infectious disease casualty militates against regarding non-state actors operating under more difficult conditions as a high-level BW threat.

Conclusion

Overall, the threat of biological attacks perpetrated by non-state actors is presently not great and should not be exaggerated. For policy-makers to assume the worst regarding the motivations and capabilities of non-state organizations might be analytically convenient and politically expedient. But, without an adequate appreciation of the preconditions for and likely effects of a non-state biological attack, governments could potentially waste a lot of effort and resources. An attack resulting in mass casualties requires that the perpetrator has a precise configuration of motivation and capability. On the basis of conceptual and empirical analysis, the characteristics of the most likely perpetrators are: a religious motivation; an apocalyptic worldview envisaging disease as a heavenly punishment; a high degree of relevant scientific expertise; and large financial resources. At present, no known non-state organization possesses a matching configuration of attributes. Aum Shinrikyo came close in the early 1990s, but its BW efforts were ultimately a failure.

In general, and for the present, non-state biological attacks should be regarded as something less than a 'mass destruction' issue, although it is important to acknowledge the possibility that crude biological agent preparations used on a small scale could nevertheless generate widespread consternation. Regarding organizations already on the radar of national intelligence agencies, the motivations for using BW are highly specific and the disincentives are many. There is some evidence that Muslim militants in Southeast Asia have taken an interest in biological agents, but it is highly unlikely that they would have the desire or resources to engage seriously in deliberate disease. For would-be perpetrators in general, there is little prospect of attracting state sponsorship. And without the highly sophisticated delivery mechanisms available from a state-run BW programme, infecting a target population would be extremely difficult. Biological agent delivery using crop dusters would generally fail to produce sufficient particles of a respirable size, and epidemiological and motivational factors militate against 'suicide sneezers' being a serious threat. The notion of *inadvertent* state sponsorship, however, is one that requires further exploration. After five years, the case of the anthrax attacks of 2001 in the United States remains unsolved, although the available evidence suggests strongly that both the perpetrator and the *B. anthracis* bacteria he or she used came from within the US defence establishment. For the present, the paucity of information regarding the perpetrator's identity and motivation leaves a conspicuous gap in the store of knowledge on BW issues.

Against the threat of biological attacks perpetrated by non-state actors, as well as the more serious threat posed by state-run BW programmes, there is a range of responses for avoiding or mitigating human damage. The next chapter assesses that some responses as more worthwhile than others, and that the most valuable are those that straddle both BW threats and infectious disease threats of natural origin.

7 Responses to the biological weapons problem

This chapter assesses responses to the problem of BW that have been or could be applied in East Asia. These generally fall into four categories: military, intelligence, legal and medical. Military responses include tactical response units, deterrence of BW-use by threat of nuclear attack and the recently-devised Proliferation Security Initiative (PSI). As a case study of intelligence challenges, this chapter focuses on the controversy surrounding the 2003 US-led invasion of Iraq. For both military and intelligence responses, the technical nature of BW generates considerable difficulties for those seeking to locate, assess and respond to a BW threat. Most importantly, assembling evidence of an offensive BW programme is complicated by the so-called 'dual use' problem – that is, elements of such a programme can also be employed for legitimate, peaceful purposes such as defensive military research and commercial vaccine production. Legal responses to the BW problem, at the domestic or international level, are generally framed in the context of the BWC. The nature of the weapons this treaty bans is such that the BWC is a creature vastly different from other disarmament treaties. Monitoring member-state compliance is more difficult than is the case regarding legal controls on nuclear and chemical materials. In addition, there is scope under the BWC to address other disease-based security challenges beyond the traditional arms-control paradigm. Of great significance to dealing with BW and other infectious disease threats via the BWC is the vexed issue of balancing non-proliferation in the interests of security against the need for biotechnology transfers to support human health and economic development.

The best and most broadly applicable approach to disease-based security challenges is through strong public health capabilities. The extent of damage from a deliberate attack or a naturally occurring outbreak event is highly dependent on the capacity of a country's public health system to identify, diagnose and treat victims, and to contain contagion. Accordingly, the two main pillars of security through public health are sensitive disease surveillance networks (local and global) and robust national health systems.

Military responses

The available military responses to the BW problem are few, and they are generally not of great value. This section assesses the limitations and problems associated with three such responses – rapid deployment of tactical response units, deterrence of BW use by threatening nuclear attack, and the interdiction of materials and equipment under the PSI.

Tactical response units

Fearing the prospect of nuclear, biological, chemical (NBC) and possibly radiological attacks, some governments in East Asia have shown an inclination to form specialist units within their military forces intended to counter the panoply of 'WMD' threats. In February 2002, South Korea's Defense Ministry launched its Chemical, Biological and Radiological Defense Command aimed at defending against an attack by North Korea. The unit includes biological detection vehicles, based on US technology, designed to identify, analyse and decontaminate a range of BW agents.[1] Japan is also aiming for functional improvement in the areas of specialist NBC personnel and equipment, particularly countermeasures against BW. Following the Tokyo sarin attacks of March 1995, the Japan Defense Agency set up chemical attack response brigades totalling 660 troops in 13 prefectures. Equipped to detect and identify chemical and biological agents, the purpose of these brigades is to warn other troops and authorities.[2]

The challenge for multi-task units of this sort is that attacks utilizing different scientific processes produce vastly different consequences. A 1999 report by the US National Academy of Sciences (NAS) highlighted how pairing off chemical weapons (CW) and BW inappropriately blurs the important scientific differences between the two. A practical consequence of this has been that the numerous US 'chem/bio' response teams are, in fact, almost entirely focused on detection, decontamination and treatment of casualties in a chemical attack scenario only.[3] Likewise, it seems to be the case that most of Japan's NBC response efforts are directed towards protection only against CW. This lack of operational emphasis on BW contingencies might in part be due to Japanese assessments that CW attacks are more likely. But it probably also reflects the reality that a biological attack is fundamentally different from a chemical attack in terms of response challenges. In November 2003, around 170 officials from the Tokyo city government and fire department participated in a role-playing drill, the premise of which was that the smallpox virus had been released in a Tokyo subway.[4] The problem with such a drill is that the participants would presumably have known that an attack of some sort was underway. In reality, the deliberate release of smallpox would likely be covert and would remain undiscovered until days or weeks later when patients began presenting symptoms at hospitals and doctors' surgeries.

Typical first responders (fire, police and ambulance) are generally not sufficient for containing the effects of a biological attack, and nor are special-ist NBC military personnel. A rapid response capability simply does not apply where, as would most likely be the case, no-one even knows a biological attack is going on. The October 2001 anthrax attacks in the United States were exceptional because the envelopes containing *B. anthracis* spores also contained letters advising the reader to take antibiotics. By contrast, when Aum Shinrikyo attempted to disperse anthrax bacteria and botulinum toxin during the early 1990s, the attacks remained unannounced and their occur-rence did not come to light until cult members faced trial several years later. Similarly, members of the Rajneesh cult did not announce in 1984 that they had sprinkled salmonella bacteria in salad bars in the Oregon town of The Dalles. Despite extensive epidemiological investigation, the source of the subsequent outbreak of food poisoning initially went unrecognized. Not until October 1985, over a year after the outbreak, did evidence emerge (in the course of an unrelated criminal investigation) that linked the event to the Rajneesh cult.[5] In a biological attack scenario, the true first responders would most likely be doctors, nurses, pathologists and other health professionals, and the speed of their response would depend on how quickly they recognized that certain symptoms and illnesses were out of the ordinary.

Deterrence by threat of nuclear attack

Within the East Asia region, China, the United States and North Korea wield strategic leverage by virtue of a nuclear weapons capability. Although such a capability has deterrence value in the face of conventional and other nuclear challenges, it probably could not deter a BW attack in the same way. On the whole, deterrence is not an option because the promise of nuclear retaliation against a BW attack is a weak threat. In practice, targets for retalia-tion could prove too obscure, and a nuclear strike to punish BW use by a state may be so disproportionate a response as to be politically indefensible.

With regard to the problem of proportionality, the 2002 US National Strategy to Combat Weapons of Mass Destruction states:

> The United States will continue to make clear that it reserves the right to respond with overwhelming force – including through resort to all of our options – to the use of WMD against the United States, our forces abroad, and friends and allies.[6]

This statement implies that the United States would respond to a BW attack with a nuclear strike. David Gompert favours a more explicit approach, arguing that the United States should 'present a threat of nuclear retaliation to deter a biological attack, which could be as deadly, and which might not be deterred by the threat of US conventional retaliation'.[7] It is uncertain, however, in what circumstances and at what point nuclear retaliation would constitute a proportionate and politically defensible response. Different biological agents can cause casualties to vastly differing extents, and the ultimate number of deaths would be highly dependent on the efficacy of the target country's healthcare system. For example, if an adversary used *C. burnetii*, a non-contagious agent that causes the incapacitating disease Q fever, the extremely low fatality rate would take away from any justification for massive lethal retaliation. A disproportionate nuclear revenge attack would become the greater of two evils. Moreover, in contrast to a nuclear strike that instantly causes a large number of deaths, the effects of a biological attack would occur gradually. Exactly how many illnesses or deaths would have to be suffered, and over what period of time, before a BW attack deserved a nuclear response?

The second part of the deterrence problem concerns credibility. The assumption underlying any discussion of nuclear weapons as a deterrence tool is that there is a BW perpetrator whose identity and location are known and against whom threats and retaliation strikes can be directed. The launch of a ballistic missile by and from a particular state, for example, would almost certainly be noticed. Assuming it were not intercepted and destroyed in flight, the absence on impact of a nuclear explosion or instant chemical effects would immediately arouse suspicions that the missile warhead had been carrying a biological payload. However, for these very reasons, ballistic missile delivery of BW is highly unlikely. According to Rex Kiziah, a long-range *cruise* missile that can be programmed to fly a circuitous route to the target can provide a state with a non-attributable method of BW attack, thus eliminating any attempt at retaliation.[8] However, even if the flight direction of a missile did not make clear its country of origin, the specific type of missile used might still provide some indication. To avoid retaliation, it is in the interests of a BW perpetrator to conceal or obscure the origin and occurrence of the attack. Absent the requirement for explosive dissemination, BW attacks are by nature silent, and the first indications would be days or weeks later when people start falling ill. By this time, it may be too late to track down and punish the perpetrator.

A second problem is that deterrence might simply not apply against a group motivated by religion and whose members believe they are carrying out the commands of their Supreme Being. For non-state actors pursuing a cleansing apocalypse, a devastating nuclear response to their biological attack might be precisely what they want to provoke.

If addressing the problem of BW is essentially about reducing the possibility of mass casualties, reliance on threats of nuclear retaliation is too dangerous a game to play. Relative to nuclear threats, BW threats are characterized by greater invisibility and unpredictability, and so the nuclear-based deterrent instrument is likely to be a blunt and ineffective one.

The Proliferation Security Initiative

The PSI, devised in late 2003, aims to prevent the proliferation of 'weapons of mass destruction', their delivery systems and related materials to 'terrorist groups' and 'states of proliferation concern'.[9] The latter are designated by PSI participants, most of whom are Western countries – Japan and Singapore are presently the only participants from the East Asia region. Non-proliferation is to be achieved by stopping the flow of prohibited weapons-related items by sea, air or land. The PSI is not explicitly aimed at North Korea but, having been accused of making clandestine shipments of drugs, counterfeit cash and missiles, the Pyongyang regime is clearly a prime target. Suspicious shipments on their way to North Korea have been intercepted in recent years. For example, in April 2003 a French-owned ship carrying 214 aluminium tubes destined for North Korea was intercepted as it entered the Suez Canal. The tubes were suspected of being gas centrifuge components for enriching uranium for nuclear weapons. The following month a ship loaded with 33 tons of sodium cyanide (a chemical precursor for making the deadly nerve agent tabun) was intercepted before reaching Pyongyang.[10]

As the PSI participant in closest proximity to North Korea, Japan's contribution is expected to involve gathering and sharing information about suspected smuggling ships, and bolstering ship inspections in Japanese territorial waters. In May 2003, Japanese authorities working with Hong Kong officials raided a Tokyo trading company, Meishin (owned by a Korean), to seize electronic equipment bound for North Korea. The company had tried to illegally export three specialized power-supply devices that could have aided North Korea's uranium enrichment programme or could have been used in missile-launch devices. Even after the raid, the same company tried to export a sensitive electronic scale to North Korea that could have been used in a BW programme,[11] although such an item could also be used for many legitimate medical or commercial purposes.

Moving beyond general concerns about 'WMD' proliferation, it is difficult to see how the PSI could offer a valuable new solution to the specific problem of BW in East Asia. To the extent that North Korea is the principal target, it is important to distinguish BW from other weapons categories. On this point, it is significant that a recent CIA report to the US Congress, while expressing concern that North Korea is a supplier of missile and possibly nuclear technology, makes no mention of Pyongyang being a supplier of BW technology.[12] North Korea might, on the other hand, be in the market for BW programme ingredients. Even so, the PSI is not a magic bullet likely to overcome the fundamental scientific difficulties associated with addressing BW threats. At the level of *tangible* proliferation, efforts to stop the spread of BW face dual-use dilemmas more profound than those that arise in relation to other weapons categories – many of the ingredients for a nuclear programme are highly specialized, and it is generally only large quantities of CW precursors that may be deemed militarily significant. By contrast, biological agents can be grown from a tiny sample quantity. And, in the unlikely event that such a thing could be intercepted in transit, it might have been intended all along for medical purposes as a reference strain for a diagnostic laboratory. In general, however, the spread of BW-relevant technology is an *intangible* phenomenon based on the knowledge and behaviour of biological scientists. As will be discussed in Part III of this book, BW 'proliferation' is predominantly about flows of scientific information rather than shipments of materials.

Intelligence responses: the case of Iraq

The science that underlies BW production and proliferation presents immense challenges for those seeking to locate, assess and respond to BW threats. Many countries could develop a BW programme using entirely their own resources, thus limiting the possibilities for interdicting imported ingredients through an arrangement like the PSI. Also, the concealment of biological-agent production facilities is relatively simple because of the technical overlap with legitimate research and commercial biotechnology. A BW facility could conceivably be located in a city and be virtually indistinguishable from other buildings even in a high-resolution satellite image. At the scientific level, in the context of the rapidly accelerating biotechnology revolution, a key challenge for intelligence agencies is to effectively monitor the sheer quantity of information being posted and exchanged on the Internet. Published advances in genetic engineering, for example, might have relevance for the future creation of pathogenic micro-organisms modified to circumvent existing vaccines or antibiotics. This in turn could have implications for responding to BW with public health measures.

In contrast to other forms of weaponry, 'capability' is an inherently vague concept when it comes to BW. Most countries could produce BW agents if they wanted to because any country with a basic fermentation industry to support commercial production of beer, yoghurt, yeast, biopesticides, vaccines or antibiotics has sufficient means to make crude preparations of basic BW agents like anthrax. Nevertheless, it seems only a small minority of countries possessing the technological capability to pursue a BW programme have actually done so. Identifying exactly which countries these are, and assessing their BW capability, is inherently difficult and the greater part of BW threat assessment involves making judgements on the basis of limited intelligence.

Where the subject of intelligence gathering and assessment is a suspected state-run BW programme, the main sources of information are programme defectors and other human intelligence sources. Physical evidence can be used to establish a country's BW capability, but assembling evidence of offensive intent necessarily requires access to inside knowledge. The drawbacks of human intelligence are that it can sometimes be vague, inaccurate or otherwise misleading. Sources may present their own assessments, suppositions and interpretations as fact, and these may actually be false. Misunderstanding by a source is a particular problem when the intelligence relates to high technology, as is often the case with BW. A source might also be seeking to advance a political agenda or may be feeding an intelligence agency disinformation.

Significant intelligence breakthroughs regarding a state's intent have resulted from defections by informed insiders. However, this was not the case prior to the 2003 US-led invasion of Iraq, when the United States relied primarily on a single source, codenamed Curveball, to assess Iraq's pre-war BW status. At no stage did US intelligence officers have direct contact with their source, whose evidence was being transmitted through a cooperative arrangement with a German intelligence agency. It was subsequently revealed in a report to the US President that Curveball had been transmitting false information and that this contributed to flawed US assessments of Iraq's military capabilities.[13]

The circumstances surrounding the US decision in 2003 to invade Iraq demonstrate that accurate intelligence about illicit BW activities is extremely difficult to obtain. The stated justification for the invasion was that Iraq allegedly possessed banned weapons in contravention of UN Security Council resolutions calling for disarmament. Once the country was under occupation, the Iraq Survey Group (ISG) was tasked with finding physical evidence that would retrospectively support this allegation. The ISG director, David Kay, issued an interim report to the US Congress in October 2003 which, to the surprise of some observers, concluded that the combined effect of sanctions, inspections and US air attacks in 1991 and 1998 had effectively destroyed Iraq's ability to produce chemical weapons after the Gulf War. He had also found no evidence that Iraq took significant steps, following the expulsion of UN weapons inspectors in 1998, to build nuclear weapons or produce fissile material.[14] Thereafter, much of the ISG's attention turned to BW.

Evidence upon which the United States relied heavily to establish Iraq's BW status was two trailers, discovered in April and May 2003, alleged to be part of a mobile BW production unit. The US hypothesis was that, by making production facilities mobile, Iraq could more easily circumvent the pre-invasion UN weapons inspection process. The significance of the trailers was the subject of intense debate within the US intelligence community, with experts divided on technical grounds over whether the trailers could actually have produced BW. At the end of May 2003, the CIA issued a report on its analysis of the trailers. The report described the results of examinations as being largely consistent with US intelligence reporting before the war. The two trailers were alleged to have been designed to produce pathogenic agents in liquid form. For this purpose, they were equipped with fermentation units, water supply tanks, a water chiller and gas collection devices. The report argued that the trailers were unlikely to have been used for legitimate purposes such as water purification, vaccine production or biopesticides. Rather, the size and nature of the equipment inside the trailers indicated that BW agent production was their only logical purpose.[15] In opposition to the report's findings, other analysts pointed out that the trailers lacked equipment for steam sterilization, normally a prerequisite for any kind of biological production. Not having such equipment available between production runs would, they argued, result in contamination and failed weapons.[16] Another theory was that the trailers were used to produce hydrogen for artillery weather balloons, although the CIA report stated that this was a cover story concocted by the Iraqis to conceal the real purpose of the trailers. Some features of one trailer – a gas collection system and the presence of a caustic substance – were consistent with both biological agent production and hydrogen production. The report argued, however, that the trailer was unnecessarily large and its equipment not suited for the efficient production of hydrogen.[17]

At the time the report on the trailers was drafted, engineering teams from the US Defense Intelligence Agency (DIA) had not concluded their own analysis. In findings leaked to the *New York Times*, it was revealed that a majority of the DIA engineers believed hydrogen production to be the true purpose of the trailers.[18] This cast doubt on the CIA report's opening claim that the trailers constituted 'the strongest evidence to date that Iraq was hiding a biological warfare program'.[19] Ultimately, the ISG assessed that 'the mobile units were impractical for biological agent production and almost certainly designed and built for the generation of hydrogen'.[20] Combined with the revelations of Curveball's fabricated evidence, the collapse of the trailer story was the fatal blow to the US case against Iraq regarding BW.

The invasion of Iraq was ostensibly intended to disarm Iraq of BW and other banned weapons allegedly in its possession. It was a radical step and one whose justification under international law is highly questionable. The likely illegality of the invasion should not, however, overshadow the array of possibilities for addressing the BW problem via legal means.

Legal responses: the Biological Weapons Convention

The first international legal attempt to limit biological warfare was the 1925 Protocol for the Prohibition of the Use in War of Asphyxiating, Poisonous or Other Gases, and of Bacteriological Methods of Warfare (the Geneva Protocol). This treaty prohibited the use of BW but not research, development, production and possession. Most countries that ratified it reserved their right to retaliate in kind, such that the Geneva Protocol became effectively a ban on first-use of BW. When the United States under President Nixon publicly renounced its offensive BW programme in 1969, it was the first time a major power had unilaterally decided to eschew an entire weapon category. The US decision gave a huge boost to the norm against BW use and thus prepared the political and moral ground for the eventual entry into force of the 1972 Convention on the Prohibition of the Development, Production and Stockpiling of Bacteriological (Biological) and Toxin Weapons and on Their Destruction.

The greatest strength of the BWC is the universality of its norm, and most domestic and international legal responses to the BW problem operate in accordance with the letter and/or spirit of this treaty. It is widely accepted in the international community that BW are abhorrent, and the norm against their use has been internalized by individuals' and nations' value systems. Although the strong norm against BW use creates a powerful stigma for potential proliferators, it nevertheless requires constant reinforcement in the face of new security challenges. In particular, there is a danger that, as a result of technological advances and/or changed international security circumstances, some political decision-makers might convince themselves and others that BW are no longer an illegitimate means of protecting national interests. Incapacitating biological agents is one area in which future advances in biotechnology might lead to new and more precise forms of 'non-lethal' BW. Bioregulators are naturally occurring chemical substances, not of themselves toxic, that operate by sending 'messages' inside the human nervous, endocrine and immune systems. These substances could be exploited for military purposes to cause non-lethal effects such as rapid unconsciousness, paralysis, hypertension or psychological disturbances.[21] For example, the July–August 2005 issue of *Military Review* contained an article entitled 'Ultramicro, nonlethal, and reversible: looking ahead to military biotechnology'.[22] The authors described and advocated the use of 'biotechnological weapons' to achieve 'nonlethal effects', but they made no mention of the BWC. In the realm of CW, the 1993 Chemical Weapons Convention (CWC) contemplates legitimate uses for chemical agents that have incapacitating effects. With regard to the BWC, however, BW are banned categorically, whether lethal or not.

Beyond the important threshold issue of the norm against BW, three key issues examined in this section are:

1   the prospects for BWC-based responses to disease-based security challenges in general;
2   the extent to which countries in East Asia have legislated to implement the Convention's provisions; and
3   the tension that exists between non-proliferation through export controls and development through technology transfers.

A new approach to the BWC

Prior to 2001, the issue attracting most political attention as a means of strengthening the BWC was a legal instrument for monitoring compliance by member states. An Ad Hoc Group (AHG) of member states had a mandate, granted at a Special Review Conference in 1994, to negotiate a verification protocol. Broadly speaking, greater confidence in treaty compliance was to be generated by:

1   declarations by member states of existing BW stockpiles and potentially BW-capable facilities;
2   routine and unannounced visits to declared or suspected BW-relevant sites; and
3   investigations of suspicious disease outbreaks.

However, the AHG negotiations were brought to an abrupt end after 2001 when the United States announced it would not support a draft protocol presented to the Fifth BWC Review Conference.

The international reaction to the US position was generally unfavourable. Nevertheless, without the support of the world's superpower, the prospects for BWC verification in the future are bleak. Until the Sixth Review Conference in 2006, the BWC member states instead undertook, in the course of three annual meetings from 2003 to 2005, to 'discuss, and promote common understanding and effective action' on:

1   national measures to implement the Convention, including penal legislation;
2   national mechanisms for security and oversight of pathogenic microorganisms and toxins;
3   enhancing international capabilities for responding to alleged use of BW or suspicious outbreaks of disease;
4   strengthening and broadening national and international mechanisms for the surveillance, detection, diagnosis and combating of infectious diseases affecting humans, animals and plants; and
5   the content, promulgation and adoption of codes of conduct for scientists.[23]

This new process for reviewing the BWC could shift the BW problem away from the traditional arms-control paradigm and towards broader notions of disease-based threats to security. For example, recent reforms of the WHO and the IHR are highly relevant to the challenge, identified in the new BWC negotiating process, of responding to infectious diseases outbreaks through national and international mechanisms. More generally, the 2003–2005 discussions could generate greater understanding of how best to address a larger array of overlapping disease-based security challenges in an era of emerging natural diseases and rapid advances in microbiology. A particular advantage of the new negotiation process is that discussions among member states may now be less about making the BWC emulate verifiable regimes governing other weapons. Whereas there are mechanisms for monitoring the CWC and the 1968 Nuclear Nonproliferation Treaty, the BWC is often characterized as the weak link in the global WMD non-proliferation regime for its lack of verification provisions. However, it is a mistake to think that addressing the problem of BW is scientifically comparable to dealing with chemical or nuclear weapons. The technical characteristics of BW are such that it was always going to be difficult to have a high degree of confidence in any system for verifying compliance with the BWC. Monitoring nuclear and chemical materials is easier because of their rarity and required volumes respectively. A few kilograms of plutonium can form the basis of a devastating nuclear weapon, and particular chemical agents acquired in sufficient quantities can be said to be militarily significant. In the context of BW, however, it makes no sense to be on the alert for specific quantities of material. This is because vast quantities of BW agent can be grown up from seed stocks of micro-organisms in a relatively short space of time.

By making the review of the BWC resemble less a quest for verification, the new process moves away from the 'WMD' paradigm and presents BW as needing to be considered in two broad dimensions. First, the nature of the BW problem is largely technological and normative rather than physical. And, second, there is substantial overlap in dealing with deliberate and natural disease outbreak events. By contrast, the challenge of nuclear and chemical weapons centres largely on physical quantities of materials, and their effects could never be compared to a natural event. In the dimension of technology and norms, arms-control mechanisms pertaining to nuclear and chemical weapons do not provide a good model for how to manage the security challenges of the new revolution in biotechnology. A vital difference is that this revolution is being driven primarily not by secretive military programmes, but rather by legitimate commercial and open academic research. Whereas the traditional arms-control approach is to contemplate weapons as physical objects stored in an arsenal, BW are better understood as a phenomenon that is mostly intangible and behavioural. In this context, the 2003–2005 BWC process focused explicitly on the people who handle pathogenic micro-organisms through topics such as the criminalization of BW activities, rules for the handling of pathogens and codes of conduct for biological scientists.

The substantial overlap between deliberate and natural disease events is brought out by international discussions on responding to alleged use of BW, and on disease surveillance and response. Here it is important to note that, in terms of the ongoing struggle between humans and pathogenic micro-organisms, the BWC was born in an era very different from the present. The opening of the Convention for signature in 1972 was preceded and facilitated by President Nixon's decision in 1969 to abandon the US offensive BW programme. In the same year, US Surgeon General William H. Steward testified before Congress that he was ready to 'close the book' on infectious disease.[24] Such optimism derived from widespread confidence that, in the developed world at least, new antibiotics and vaccines would bring about a lasting human victory over pathogenic micro-organisms. By contrast, the BWC today has to operate in an era of emerging and re-emerging infectious diseases. As such, the Convention is most usefully seen not as part of a 'WMD' non-proliferation regime, but rather as part of an expanded response to disease-based security threats in general.

Relevant to the future role of the BWC, there are still important issues to be addressed regarding the Convention in its current form. The following sections examine the extent to which BWC prohibitions are part of the domestic law of countries in East Asia, and the tension generated by the Convention's dual objectives of non-proliferation and technology transfer.

National implementing legislation: a survey of East Asia

Article IV of the BWC requires each member state to adopt appropriate legal measures to ensure that the treaty's fundamental prohibitions regarding BW, contained in Article I, are enforceable under national law throughout its territory. This section provides a survey of BWC legislation as it has been implemented by countries in East Asia. The information is derived from statements by country representatives at BWC meetings and from a database of implementation legislation prepared by the London-based Verification Research, Training and Information Centre (VERTIC). In addition, indications of the nature and extent of national BWC implementation may be gleaned from country reports lodged in accordance with UN Security Council Resolution (UNSCR) 1540. Adopted on 28 April 2004, this Resolution requires all UN member states to refrain from providing any support to non-state actors that attempt to acquire nuclear, chemical and biological weapons.

In the cases of Taiwan and North Korea, it is difficult to discern through public sources what measures are in place to govern pathogenic agents and related equipment. Taiwanese legislation is not included in any BWC-oriented lists because Taiwan is not diplomatically eligible to join the UN or the BWC. In the case of North Korea, which is party to the Convention, VERTIC was unable to identify any relevant legislation to enforce its provisions.[25] This is not of itself cause for alarm – when VERTIC conducted its survey, it acknowledged that many countries likely did not provide advice on domestic legislation because of translation issues or a lack of administrative staff to carry out such a task.[26] On the other hand, North Korea is governed by a military dictatorship rather than the rule of law, so there are grounds for concern that BW-relevant materials and equipment might not be subject to adequate controls. And, although North Korea, as a UN member state, is required to lodge a report on implementation of UNSCR 1540, it had not done so as of late-2006.[27] South Korea, by contrast, has recently enacted BW-relevant legislation relating to export controls and counterterrorism. Other laws are in place, dating back to the 1950s and 1960s, to deal with plant, animal and human contagious diseases.[28] In addition, South Korea has stated its intention to enact a special law 'prescribing the reporting and inspection of manufacturing and production facilities of biological weapons-related materials with a view to establishing a comprehensive and systematic control and management system'.[29]

China has instituted a number of laws and regulations to prevent the non-peaceful use of biological agents and related technologies. It also has legislation to deal with naturally occurring disease threats. The relevant areas include criminal law, import licensing, export controls, customs, quarantine, prevention and control of infectious diseases, responses to public health emergencies (for example, measures for reporting, controlling and treating SARS), and biological safety including facility construction and storage of bacteria species.[30] Of direct relevance to UNSCR 1540, Amendment III of the Criminal Law of the People's Republic of China prohibits persons or entities from manufacturing, acquiring, possessing, storing, transporting, transferring or using BW, as well as financing and assisting such activities.[31]

When Japan ratified the BWC in 1982, the Japanese Diet enacted the BWC Implementing Law. Using the language of Articles I and III of the Convention, the Law criminalizes the development, production, stockpiling and transfer of BW. It also empowers relevant ministers to order persons to make compulsory reports regarding their activities to the extent necessary for preventing activities with biological agents that serve no peaceful purpose.[32] More recently, under the 2002 'Act on Punishment of Financing to offences of public intimidation', Japan has outlawed the financing of a 'terrorist act which is related to biological weapons'.[33]

Brunei implements the BWC through a stand-alone piece of legislation, the Biological Weapons Act 1975, which 'prohibits any person from developing, producing, stockpiling, acquiring or retaining any biological agent or toxin of a certain type contrary to peaceful purposes'.[34] Malaysia, by contrast, has not found it necessary to enact new legislation to implement its BWC obligations. Relevant legislative provisions exist in its Corrosive and Explosive Substances and Offensive Weapons Act 1958, the Arms Act 1960, the Customs Act 1967, and the Prevention and Control of Infectious Diseases Act 1988. In addition, the Malaysian Penal Code criminalizes 'any unlawful or negligent or malignant act which is likely to spread infection of any disease dangerous to life'.[35] Nevertheless, according to its UNSCR 1540 report to the UN, 'Malaysia is currently studying the need to draft a specific law to implement more effectively the BWC'.[36]

In Cambodia, Article 54 of the Constitution prohibits the manufacturing, use and storage of nuclear, chemical and biological weapons. Cambodia also has laws requiring authorization from the Minister for Health for production, trade, import and export of pharmaceuticals.[37] Laos has no existing BW-relevant legal framework, although as of May 2005 it was 'in a process of amending its Penal Law which will cover crime of terrorist acts involving the use of nuclear, chemical and biological weapons'.[38] In Indonesia, Law no. 15/2003 on Eradication of Criminal Acts of Terrorism criminalizes the acquisition, possession, transfer and use of BW, and the government has 'identified the urgency' of having stand-alone legislation with respect to BW.[39] And in Singapore, the parliament passed a new Biological Agents and Toxins Bill in October 2005. The legislation, introduced against the backdrop of an increase in the number of Singaporean institutions working with pathogenic micro-organisms, regulates the possession, use, import, transfer and transportation of 93 biological agents.[40]

Vietnam has import/export and penal laws governing toxic substances, but none specifically directed to BW,[41] whereas Thailand has a range of BW-relevant laws in place that require licences to import/export certain goods and that allow for prohibition of the transfer of such goods. These include the Disease Control Act 1980, the Hazardous Substance Act 1992, and the Pathogens and Toxins Act 2001. Moreover, Thailand stated in November 2004 that it would update national control lists for dual-use items and implement stricter controls over the import of biological substances.[42] As of late-2006, Timor-Leste had not lodged a UNSCR 1540 return, and those returns lodged by Myanmar (not a BWC member state) and the Philippines contained no information on BW-relevant laws.

To the extent that BWC-relevant laws are in place around East Asia, they play an important role in strengthening the norm against BW and reducing the likelihood of biological attacks. However, US experience suggests that those seeking to enforce such laws in the aftermath of an attack are likely to encounter considerable forensic challenges – more than five years after the 2001 anthrax envelope attacks in the United States, the perpetrator has yet to be identified and punished.

Export controls and technology transfers

Article X of the BWC requires member states to 'facilitate . . . the fullest possible exchange of equipment, materials, and scientific and technological information for the use of bacteriological (biological) agents and toxins for peaceful purposes' and to 'cooperate in contributing with other states . . . to the further development or application of scientific discoveries in the field of bacteriology (biology) for prevention of disease, or for other peaceful purposes'. The language of Article X (specifically, 'for peaceful purposes') is such that the provision is subject to interpretations of intent. This inevitably generates a tension with Article III of the Convention under which member states undertake 'not to transfer to any recipient whatsoever . . . any of the agents, toxins, weapons, equipment or means of delivery specified in Article I'. Indeed, it is one of the greatest elements of international distrust on BW issues that developed countries are afraid to share biotechnology with developing countries for fear that it will not be used 'for peaceful purposes'. Herein lies the dilemma of how to achieve the Convention's dual objectives of non-proliferation and technology transfer. This section explores the general issues at stake in contemplating the sharing of infectious-disease-relevant biotechnology and concludes with a discussion of how these issues are perceived by certain countries in East Asia.

Export controls on dual-use technology, materials and equipment are the primary means by which developed countries, through an organization known as the Australia Group (AG), pursue BW (and CW) non-proliferation. The AG maintains a series of lists that define dual-use precursor chemicals, biological agents, chemical and biological equipment, and related technology. Participating states are informally committed to ensure these items are subject to national export controls, and they assess export licence applications in accordance with an agreed set of guidelines.[43] Advocates of export controls generally do not pretend that these are an adequate response to BW proliferation. Rather, export controls are seen as an interim measure that buys time until a better approach emerges. The main criticism directed at export controls is that they discriminate against developing countries by restricting access to vital technology transfers. For example, the AG has been criticized for maintaining a 'warning list' of chemicals not to be exported to certain countries that differs from and extends the lists of chemicals in Schedules to the CWC. Fears have been expressed in the past that this practice could extend to the BWC.[44] However, there appears to have been a recent softening of the traditional criticisms levelled against the AG. Related to this, some non-AG countries have recognized the value of the Group's comprehensive control lists by adopting similar lists of their own to prevent the proliferation of chemical and biological weapons-relevant technology and equipment.[45]

The sharing of biotechnology between developed and developing countries is a vexed issue in negotiations to make the BWC work more effectively. From one point of view, pursuing non-proliferation through export controls only aggravates international tensions. The alternative perspective is that to allow too liberal an approach on the transfer of biotechnology is to make BW use more likely. For over 30 years, since the BWC was opened for signature, the question of how to implement Article X has been largely intractable. Nevertheless, it is possible that new security considerations could see a shift in non-proliferation policies which, by their very nature, tend to pit possessors of certain technologies against non-possessors. Biotechnology could become a special case because of disease-based threats that extend beyond the problem of BW. In particular, the primary and ongoing infectious disease concern of most countries is controlling natural outbreaks and not the possibility of a BW attack.

Within East Asia there are mixed attitudes to the issue of export controls and technology transfers, and this is largely a reflection of the region's mix of developed and developing countries. Japan, one of the world's largest investors in biotechnology research and development, believes firmly in non-proliferation through export controls and is a participant in the AG. In the spirit of Article X, however, it has provided development assistance to developing countries bilaterally or through international organizations in fields including biotechnology. For example, Japan has organized seminars, offered training programmes for researchers and improved the capabilities of research institutions in such countries.[46] South Korea, also an AG participant, has actively participated in international exchanges of scientific and technological information relating to the use of biological agents and toxins for peaceful purposes. It has also provided assistance to countries in need of advice on disease control and health issues generally. For example, the International Vaccine Institute, headquartered in Seoul, is an institution devoted to strengthening the capacity of developing countries in the development, production and use of vaccines in immunization programmes.[47]

China attaches great importance to its development and progress in the biological field and has stated its desire for more cooperation and exchange among BWC member states in the peaceful use of biotechnology.[48] Excluded from the AG, Beijing regards as discriminatory export control groups created by mainly Western countries that establish a monopoly on certain forms of technology. Such regimes, it argues, serve to deepen resentment among excluded countries and undermine international cooperation by using non-proliferation as a pretext. China believes the AG must be replaced by national export controls coordinated through mechanisms developed within the framework of a BWC verification regime.[49] To demonstrate China's sincerity in this belief, a 2002 statement by the Chinese Foreign Ministry detailed:

1   China's Regulations on Export Control of Dual-Use Biological Agents and Related Equipment and Technologies; and
2   its Dual-Use Biological Agents and Related Equipment and Technologies Control List.

The Regulations, in force as of December 2002, contain measures to strengthen export controls to prevent diversion of dual-use biological agents, related equipment and technologies towards production of BW. Domestic measures include an export licensing system, licence application process and criminal prosecution for violations. The Regulations also cover the receiving party and require guarantees that biological materials will not be diverted towards weapon production and unapproved third parties. The Control List, updated in mid-2006, sets out pathogens covered by the Regulations, and it also covers dual-use equipment such as containment facilities used to conduct research on pathogenic micro-organisms, protective equipment, fermentation units and aerosol inhalation chambers.[50] At the same time, the contents of this control list reveal that China objects to the AG export control regime only in principle and not in practice. In the scope of its controls on 79 pathogen types and seven broad categories of dual-use equipment and related technologies, the Chinese list is 'basically the same as that of the Australia Group'.[51]

Indonesia regards biotechnology as an important means of advancing human welfare and strongly advocates the full implementation of Article X. It is anxious that the BWC should not hamper the use, research and development of biological agents for peaceful purposes, particularly in addressing infectious diseases that occur in tropical countries. At the Fifth BWC Review Conference in 2001, the head of the Indonesian delegation stated that 'technical and scientific cooperation is important not only for the socio-economic development of the developing countries, but also for fighting infectious diseases and effectively countering the current threat of bio-terrorism'.[52] This statement implied strongly that export controls on disease-relevant biotechnology and related equipment potentially hinder medical advancements and public health responses in some countries.

Other barriers for developing countries trying to address naturally occurring disease threats include, for example, international rules governing intellectual property. These arguably reduce the capacity of some developing countries to supply their people with affordable healthcare. In particular, the World Trade Organization's 1994 agreement on Trade-Related Aspects of Intellectual Property Rights affords 20 years of worldwide patent protection to technological inventions, including vaccines and medicines. Through patenting, a pharmaceutical company that develops a new drug enjoys a temporary global monopoly on all production, pricing and marketing of that patented drug. In the context of a looming influenza pandemic, the Swiss pharmaceutical company Roche has demonstrated its preparedness to issue extra licences for producing antiviral drugs. This illustrates the extent to which corporations as well as governments need to be engaged in facilitating the transfer of biotechnology to help developing countries fight infectious disease threats.

Drug supplies are but one issue when seeking to address disease-based security challenges through strong public health capabilities. As a response applicable to both BW and naturally occurring disease threats, public health is the most worthwhile area in which to invest financial resources and political attention. Whether an outbreak is of deliberate or natural origin, the extent of damage is highly dependent on the capacity of national, international and global health systems to identify, diagnose and treat victims, and to contain contagion.

Public health responses: biological weapons and natural plagues

Many of the basic measures needed to protect populations against emerging infectious diseases – for example, syndromic surveillance, diagnostics and medical therapies – are the same as would be required to thwart or mitigate a BW attack. Chinese communist leader Mao Zedong recognized this in 1952 when, amidst the controversy over alleged US involvement in biological warfare during the Korean War, he launched China's first Patriotic Hygiene Campaign. The slogan for the campaign was: 'Mobilise to promote hygiene, to reduce disease, to raise the level of the people's health, and to smash the germ warfare of the American imperialists!'[53] Given the overlap between health and security needs, a 'dual-use' response is the most worthwhile approach to BW threats. Because the magnitude of the BW problem is so difficult to calculate, and the intention of potential attackers so hard to gauge, it makes sense to focus on broadly applicable remedies aimed at limiting vulnerability to outbreak events. The result of such a focus would be to improve public health in general, regardless of whether biological attacks ever occurred. For these reasons, policy-makers may find that public health responses to the BW threat are more politically defensible than other responses requiring comparable expenditure.

The two main pillars of security through public health are sensitive and well-connected infectious disease surveillance networks (local and global) and robust national health systems. In addition to addressing ongoing human welfare imperatives, these pillars serve three important security functions:

1   they may lead potential BW perpetrators to suppose that the effects of an attack would be thwarted or at least reduced;
2   they directly address human vulnerability to the effects of a successful BW attack; and
3   most importantly, they serve also to bolster defences against disease outbreaks of natural origin.

As the first part of this book has already assessed disease surveillance and other public health measures in the context of naturally occurring infectious disease threats, this section focuses on the value of such measures as responses to BW threats specifically.

An important point of difference is that the dread which attaches to particular infectious diseases, combined with the ghastly notion of a fellow human perpetrator, would arguably generate adverse psychological effects beyond what might be expected during an outbreak event of natural origin. In the event of a BW attack, an early public health challenge would be to deal with uninfected individuals who were misattributing symptoms of fear to biological agents and overwhelming healthcare facilities. One estimate is that, following a chemical or biological incident thought to be deliberately caused, for every one person seeking hospital care for physical injuries, at least six would present with psychological concerns.[54] India's experience of an outbreak event involving plague well illustrates the adverse impact of dread on public health responses. Between 26 August and 5 October 1994, 5,150 suspected cases of pneumonic or bubonic plague were reported in eight Indian states. Around 600,000 people fled the city of Surat in one night, and vital medical personnel were among them. In Delhi, 1,200 kilometres away, hospitals were flooded. Adding to the general panic was an unsubstantiated rumour that neighbouring Pakistan had deliberately introduced genetically-engineered *Y. pestis* bacteria that it had acquired from the former Soviet Union. Ultimately, there were only 167 confirmed plague cases and 53 deaths.[55] But the deep dread of plague, a disease with a dark history, generated damage and disruption vastly disproportionate to the amount of illness and death that resulted from this outbreak event.

In order to reduce the 'value-added' dread factor associated with BW-generated outbreaks (actual or suspected), and to mitigate the amount of damage they cause, it is necessary to maintain strong public health capabilities at the national and international levels. Most important are those capabilities that relate to disease surveillance and the treatment of patients.

Disease surveillance and response

Because a biological agent takes time to incubate inside a victim's body, it may be days or weeks before the symptoms of a deliberate disease attack become apparent. Post-infection detection of a BW attack would happen when cases of disease were diagnosed simultaneously in multiple surgeries, clinics and hospitals. But without adequate networks for communication and reporting, nobody would know a disease outbreak was going on or the extent to which it had spread. With highly sensitive systems for disease surveillance in place, outbreaks of deadly, contagious, long-incubating diseases could be detected and contained rapidly wherever in the world they occurred. Enhancing disease surveillance sensitivity requires, for example, training clinicians to recognize the signs and symptoms of BW-relevant diseases they would not normally encounter in their medical practices. It also requires expanded diagnostic capacity worldwide to ensure existing laboratories are not swamped with samples of suspected BW agents.

An increase in illness associated with a BW attack would be more difficult to detect if it occurred during a seasonal surge in naturally occurring infectious disease. For this reason, the WHO emphasizes the importance of routine surveillance for emerging diseases and those prone to epidemics. This would enhance the capacity of public health authorities to detect and investigate deliberately caused outbreaks; an unusual event would be more easily recognized in the light of background data on the natural behaviour of infectious diseases. Such data includes the disease's geographical and seasonal occurrence, and the characteristic epidemiological, demographic and clinical features of an outbreak.[56] Although the WHO encourages disease surveillance to detect suspicious outbreaks and provides advice to its member states on national BW preparedness and response programmes, it would not be appropriate for this organization to investigate allegations of BW use. The December 2004 report of the UN High-Level Panel on Threats, Challenges and Change recommended that the UN Security Council consult the WHO Director-General 'to establish the necessary procedures for working together in the event of a suspicious or overwhelming [natural] outbreak of infectious disease'.[57]

This recommendation, clearly aimed at garnering greater resources and authority for dealing with outbreak events, nevertheless did not recognize the political distinction that may be drawn between an 'overwhelming natural outbreak' and one designated as 'suspicious'. Resources and responses flow differently depending on whether a situation touches the humanitarian or the security nerve of governments and non-government organizations. If WHO resources were used to investigate a politically motivated accusation of BW use, for example, there is a danger that this would compromise the organization's humanitarian objectives. To a great extent, the access and goodwill accorded the WHO is dependent on its reputation as a neutral, scientific body. Too close an association with the UN Security Council might make some countries reluctant to cooperate with WHO investigations. An alternative for dealing with suspicious outbreaks might be to establish a separate pool of investigators organized under the auspices of the BWC. In any case, the response role of the WHO, an organization without vast resources of its own, would be in the areas of international coordination and expert advice. The rallying points for the core business of treating patients during an out-break event are national health systems.

Health system surge capacity

In the event of a biological attack, a strong national health system could quickly be alerted to the nature and extent of the problem, could treat and contain the number of patients, and generally restore the health confidence of the target population. Unfortunately, health system infrastructures in virtually all countries are under-resourced. Hospital staff, facilities, supplies and equipment are usually stretched to the limit on day-to-day matters and generally cannot cope well with small, sudden surges in patient numbers. A key response to BW is therefore to build a surge capacity into the health system to allow for outbreak contingencies. Emergency plans would be needed in areas such as staff protection, patient triage on a mass scale, distributing and administering drug and other therapy, and coordination with relevant national and international agencies. Of particular importance is the surge capacity of diagnostic laboratories. Rapidly establishing a diagnosis is critical for public health response purposes because this then guides the use of vaccines, drugs and other medical interventions. A study published in *Nature* in December 2004 predicted that 67 to 76 per cent of victims from a biological attack using anthrax bacteria would not become ill if they began taking antibiotics within six days of exposure and continued to take them for at least 60 days. However, if antibiotics were not administered until ten days after exposure, less than 50 per cent of victims would be prevented from falling ill.[58]

Measures to establish a health system surge capacity might well be resisted by national governments intent on cutting costs in the health sector. And, in the context of BW threats, it might be unrealistic to expect public health agencies to allocate resources to improve emergency preparedness from within their existing budgets – a BW attack might never happen, whereas hospitals face life-threatening illnesses of natural origin every day. Similarly, the threat of emerging, fast-spreading diseases like SARS, although more predictable than a BW attack, is for many countries not as obvious and immediate a threat as heart disease and cancer. The threat of BW alone probably cannot win policy priority and added resources, and nor can that of naturally occurring infectious disease outbreaks. Dealing with the first might be seen as too expensive a commitment for a security threat that might never materialize and whose credibility is contestable, and the second could continue to be regarded purely as a health issue. In combination, however, the threats of deliberate and natural disease create a dual imperative for governments and other relevant entities to improve public health capabilities. First, extra expenditure on security grounds to resist BW would be more justifiable financially because it also promises to improve defences against naturally occurring diseases. And, second, extra expenditure on health grounds to resist natural infectious disease threats would be more acceptable politically because its direct applicability to BW threats adds a compelling security element.

Conclusion

The responses that have been or could be employed in East Asia to address the problem of BW are of varying worth. To illustrate the general weakness of military responses, this chapter identified the shortcomings of tactical response units, nuclear-based deterrence of BW use and the PSI. This is not to suggest, however, that military personnel and resources are irrelevant. During an outbreak event of deliberate or natural origin, they could play an important supportive role in areas such as maintaining civil order and ensuring the security of medical supplies and facilities. Regarding intelligence responses, the potential dual-use nature of BW-related agents, equipment and facilities means that accurate intelligence, much less evidence, about illicit activities is extremely hard to obtain. This is well demonstrated by the failure of the United States to produce evidence that its pre-Iraq War claims of Iraqi BW possession were correct.

Legal responses to BW are generally framed by reference to the BWC. The Convention embodies the longstanding international norm against deliberate disease, although it requires constant reinforcement in the face of new political and security challenges. The establishment of a protocol for verifying compliance with the BWC seems to be a lost cause, although such an instrument was probably not well-suited to addressing the BW problem in any case. The advantage of the new negotiation process that emerged out of the Fifth BWC Review Conference is that discussions among member states appear now to be less about making the Convention emulate verifiable regimes governing other weapons. Rather, the Convention could more usefully become part of an expanded response to disease-based security threats in general.

In the context of East Asia, the two BWC issues of most concern are the extent of national implementation of relevant legislation and the tension that exists between the Convention's dual objectives of non-proliferation and technology transfer. Regional implementation of BWC laws and regulations is patchy, and outright gaps in legal coverage could hinder the ability of some countries to prevent or respond to a biological attack. However, it is important to acknowledge that, for developing countries especially, the most pressing infectious disease threats are those of natural origin. The need for access to biotechnology that might address ongoing health challenges is one reason why countries such as Indonesia and China favour the full implementation of Article X of the BWC. With Japan and South Korea having elected to pursue security and non-proliferation through export controls, this is a potential source of regional tension.

Of all the responses to BW, the most direct and worthwhile are those related to public health. A strong and effective public health response would be based on two main pillars. First, highly sensitive and well-connected systems for disease surveillance and response would be a vital means of containing an outbreak in its early stages and facilitating the timely treatment of victims. And, second, national health systems with surge capacity in areas such as diagnostics and patient care would be better able to cope with sudden outbreak contingencies. The added virtue of maintaining strong public health measures to respond to BW is that these are equally important for mitigating damage from naturally occurring outbreak events. The effectiveness of public health measures is vitally supported by research on pathogenic micro-organisms. Experiments that explore the properties of pathogens have the potential to reveal or enhance medical and public health responses during outbreak events, whether of deliberate or natural origin. For example, the rapid genotyping in early 2003 of the virus that causes SARS helped in the development of appropriate strategies for containment, illness management and prevention of secondary disease transmission. However, microbiology laboratories also have the potential themselves to be sources of disease-based security threats. These are explored in Part III.

Part III
Pathogen research

8 Beyond biosafety

The security consciousness of scientists

In the realm of pathogen research, control and oversight fall into two inter-related categories. The first, biosafety, is about measures and procedures for protecting the health and safety of people working in laboratories and preventing the accidental release of pathogens into the environment. The second category, biosecurity, concerns measures for preventing theft and illegal use of pathogens, such as for the production of BW. Laboratories around the world have undertaken biosafety measures for decades. By contrast, the notion of biosecurity is relatively new, having arisen mainly because of concerns about the deliberate misuse of pathogenic micro-organisms.

Biosafety and biosecurity are important issues in East Asia because investment in biotechnology is assuming greater significance in the region's economies, bringing with it more scientists and laboratories to support pathogen research. For example, Indonesia plans to expand its existing biotechnology infrastructure to include three Inter-University Centres on Biotechnology as well as numerous research facilities and culture collections. The Malaysian government has invested US$26 million to build three institutes in the new BioValley Malaysia, a large complex that is part of a plan to attract US$10 billion in biotechnology investment within a decade. The South Korean government envisages total investment in biotechnology to reach US$15 billion by 2007, while the Chinese biotechnology sector has been estimated to be growing at over 15 per cent annually. And, in 2001, Singapore embarked on a 15-year, US$8.2 billion plan to make Singapore a high-technology hub with a strong focus on biotechnology – the plan includes the US$500 million BioPolis complex.[1]

The first section of this chapter outlines the basics of laboratory safety and containment, examines the lessons from three accidental infections involving the SARS virus, and assesses biosafety in East Asia. The section on the security consciousness of biological scientists examines the circumstances of the 2001 anthrax envelope attacks in the United States, the US experience with domestic biosecurity laws and the state of biosecurity regulation in East Asia. The third section explores the security significance of so-called 'experiments of concern' and the importance of codes of conduct for scientists.

Laboratory biosafety: preventing accidental outbreaks

When dealing with a dangerous pathogen, safe laboratory practices and appropriate levels of physical containment are important measures for avoiding an accidental outbreak event. Such an event may occur in the context of research aimed at improving human health, or in the context of a programme for deliberately causing disease. An infamous example of the latter is the 1979 outbreak of inhalation anthrax (the largest such outbreak ever documented) that occurred in the former Soviet Union. A non-intentional release of agents from a BW facility in Sverdlovsk, following a failure to activate air filters early on the morning of 3 April 1979, resulted in the windborne spread of an aerosol of *B. anthracis* bacteria – at least 77 cases and 66 deaths were reported.[2]

Physically, biosafety is about placing barriers or filters between a pathogen and the researcher, and between the laboratory and the environment. Accordingly, there are two categories of containment: primary (safety equipment) and secondary (facility design). Primary barriers against exposure to infectious agents include: good laboratory practice and technique; protective gloves and coats; respirators and face shields; and sealed biological safety cabinets. The kind of secondary barriers required depends upon the risk of transmission of specific agents (see Table 8.1). Laboratories working with less hazardous agents should have sinks available, and windows fitted with fly screens. And, in laboratories where containment is more important, there should be specialized air filters and fans that generate negative atmospheric pressure – any containment breach would cause air to flow into, rather than out of, a facility.

Table 8.1 Levels of biosafety

Biosafety level	Description
BSL-1	Suitable for work with agents not known to cause disease in healthy humans. Minimal potential hazard to laboratory workers and the environment.
BSL-2	Suitable for work involving agents of moderate potential hazard to personnel and the environment.
BSL-3	Suitable for work with infectious agents that may cause serious or lethal disease as a result of exposure by inhalation, but against which vaccines and/or therapies are available.
BSL-4	Suitable for work with dangerous and exotic agents that pose a high risk of life-threatening disease, and which may be transmitted by aerosol and for which there is no vaccine or therapy available.

Source: CDC, *Laboratory Biosafety Level Criteria* (CDC Online, 30 November 2000). Online, available at: www.cdc.gov/od/ohs/biosfty/bmbl4/bmbl4s3.htm (accessed 12 June 2005).

A high level of containment does not, however, eliminate the risk of accidents. In 2004, two scientists working in BSL-4 laboratories, one American and one Russian, became infected with Ebola virus after accidentally sticking themselves with a syringe.[3] And in the United States, plans to expand the number of high-containment laboratories have generated fears that this will result in more laboratory-acquired infections and accidental releases of pathogens into the environment.[4]

Three SARS accidents

For the East Asia region, where the extent of research on pathogenic micro-organisms is also expanding, the risk of accidents occurring is similarly a concern. After the SARS outbreak of 2003 ended, laboratory-acquired SARS infections in Singapore, Taiwan and China could have produced subsequent outbreaks – all were the result of poor biosafety practices.

In September 2003, a 27-year-old postgraduate medical student working in a laboratory at the National University of Singapore (NUS) was infected with SARS. The patient was isolated in hospital after developing a fever, and later recovered. No secondary cases arose from this infection.[5] An epidemiological investigation found that inappropriate laboratory safety standards and a cross-contamination of West Nile virus samples with SARS virus in the NUS laboratory led to the infection.[6] At the request of the Singaporean government, an 11-member team, including WHO biosafety experts, was assembled to investigate equipment and procedures at all Singaporean facilities housing BSL-3 laboratories. At three out of the four facilities, the team found evidence of biosafety shortcomings. The training of laboratory workers at Singapore's Environmental Health Institute was found to be insufficient and the investigation team recommended the implementation of a good record-keeping policy. At Singapore General Hospital, there was a mixing of BSL-2 and BSL-3 activities that prejudiced good safety practices. And, at NUS, limited space and overcrowding were revealed as chronic problems, and the investigating team recommended the development of a practical safety culture among scientists and students.[7]

Lax laboratory safety procedures were also to blame when, on 17 December 2003, a medical researcher (Lieutenant Colonel Chan) in Taiwan tested positive for SARS. Working in a laboratory at the National Defence University's Institute of Preventive Medicine, Chan had been screening antiviral drugs for effectiveness against SARS. He was working in a BSL-4 laboratory in which virus samples were handled within a closed cabinet using attached gloves. Attached to the cabinet was a chamber for transporting waste materials to a sterilization unit. On 6 December, Chan noted that some liquid waste had spilled into the transportation chamber but he could not reach it using the attached gloves. He sprayed the area with alcohol and waited ten minutes. Presuming disinfection had been successful, Chan then opened the chamber to finish cleaning up the spill. That action exposed him to the

SARS virus. Chan attended a conference in Singapore the following day and developed a fever on 10 December 2003 after returning to Taiwan. On 16 December, he was admitted to hospital and the next day it was confirmed he had SARS. A total of 90 people who had been in close contact with him in Singapore and Taiwan were quarantined. Fortunately, at the time he was travelling, he did not pass the disease on to anyone because he was asymptomatic and not infectious. There was no outbreak and Chan recovered. His infection was blamed on poor safety procedures at the laboratory in which he worked.[8]

The laboratory-acquired infections resulting from accidents in Singapore and Taiwan did not result in spread beyond the affected workers. By contrast, in April 2004, China narrowly avoided another major SARS outbreak after the virus escaped from a laboratory at the Beijing Institute for Virology. On 7 March 2004, a 26-year-old medical student (Ms Song) began studying at the Institute. She and a fellow student (Mr Yang) were in a laboratory that handled samples of the SARS coronavirus. Ms Song finished her studies on 22 March and the next day travelled by train back to her home in Anhui Province. Three days later she developed a fever and afterwards returned by train to Beijing for treatment. On 29 March she was admitted to hospital as a pneumonia patient. For some reason, on 2 April, Ms Song was transferred by train to a hospital in Anhui where her mother (Mrs Wei) was most often by her side. The mother developed a fever on 8 April and died 11 days later. Meanwhile, Mr Yang had developed a fever on 17 April. Chinese health officials classified Ms Song and Mr Yang as suspected SARS patients along with Ms Li, one of the nurses who had cared for Ms Song in Beijing. Ms Li's father, mother, aunt and roommate fell ill as well.[9]

The Beijing Institute for Virology was closed and its 270 employees quarantined along with more than 700 others who may have come into contact with suspected SARS cases. The incident reached a critical juncture on 1 May 2004, the beginning of a week-long vacation in China when millions of people would start moving around the country. The concern was that, if SARS was out there, this mass movement could spark outbreaks throughout China. The government increased health screenings at airports and train stations to prevent a wider spread of the disease, and anyone with a fever was prohibited from travelling.[10] After Beijing confirmed that two patients had SARS, the government in neighbouring Taiwan responded by tightening the monitoring of travellers from the mainland.[11] Fortunately, the outbreak was limited to eight cases of illness in Beijing and Anhui Province and one death. A report issued by the Chinese Ministry of Health blamed the outbreak on a series of flaws at the Beijing Institute for Virology. A batch of supposedly inactivated SARS virus had been brought from its BSL-3 storage location into a regular laboratory (with lower safety standards), where Ms Song and Mr Yang were working on diarrhoeal viruses. The process for inactivating the virus (adding a mix of detergents) had not worked properly,[12] thus laying the ground for an accidental outbreak event.

Biosafety in East Asia

The three SARS accidents of 2003–2004 demonstrate that biosafety is a real concern in East Asia in terms of resisting disease-based security challenges. Under slightly different circumstances, each could have triggered effects comparable to a BW attack or a natural infectious disease outbreak. Individual scientific institutions in East Asia may choose to adhere to international biosafety guidelines for professional and scientific reasons, but a number of countries have taken the added step of incorporating biosafety principles into national regulations. For example, the Malaysian Penal Code criminalizes 'any unlawful or *negligent* or malignant act which is likely to spread the infection of any disease dangerous to life' (emphasis added).[13] And, in Indonesia, biosafety measures are regulated by 'the Decision of the Department of Health on the Safety in Microbiological Laboratory and Biomedics'.[14] However, the best examples of a comprehensive national commitment to biosafety in East Asia are provided by Japan, China and Singapore.

In Japan the standard for biosafety is set by the National Institute of Infectious Disease. In 1981 the Institute established the Laboratory Safety Regulation for Biological Agents. This regulation has been revised several times to take into account the WHO *Laboratory Biosafety Manual* and the biosafety systems of other countries, and it is widely referred to by other research institutes, businesses and universities in Japan as a model for biosafety management guidelines. The regulation lists pathogens to be controlled and divides them into four biohazard levels. It also prescribes safety standards for equipment and laboratory management, emergency measures, and healthcare and safety training for personnel handling biological agents.[15] Japan does not have a separate law that defines safety standards and physical protection requirements for facilities that store pathogens; however, certain standards and requirements are set forth in other laws. An example is the Pharmaceutical Affairs Law that requires pharmaceutical production facilities using pathogens to meet plant and equipment standards to prevent the leakage of pathogens. In addition, Japan's Guidelines for Recombinant DNA Experiments (established in 1979 and revised in 2002) contain detailed requirements for containment methods and equipment, transport and post-experiment disposal of genetically modified micro-organisms, and healthcare and training of personnel who conduct experiments.[16]

In China, regulatory coverage on biosafety matters is extensive. The 1986 Regulations on the Storage and Administration of Microbial Bacteria Species set out procedures for the 'separation, selection, collection, storage, identification, indexing, supplying and exchange' of bacteria species. China's Law on the Prevention and Control of Infectious Diseases (adopted in February 1989) and its Implementation Regulations (promulgated in December 1991) establish three categories of infectious bacteria and viruses based on toxicity and the seriousness of the diseases they cause. The law also administers the use, storage and transportation of such micro-organisms.[17] In 2004, following the laboratory-acquired SARS infection at the Beijing Institute of Virology, revisions to this law included new biosafety requirements – disease-control agencies, medical laboratories, or research bodies must manage virus samples correctly, and violations that lead to the spread of any disease could lead to criminal punishment.[18] In addition, the Regulations of Labor Protection in Workplaces Where Toxic Substances Are Used (promulgated in April 2002) prescribe safety measures related to facilities, equipment, health of personnel, handling and transport of toxic substances, accountability, licensing and accreditation. China's General Guidelines on Biological Safety in Microbial and Medical Laboratory (promulgated in December 2002) establish detailed requirements for the administration and design of laboratories designated BSL-2 and above, and the handling of pathogens therein, so as to prevent laboratory-acquired infections and leakage into the environment.[19]

With laws such as these in place, there remains the question of the degree to which biosafety is in fact being enhanced. In October 2005 a government survey of 8,000 medical and research facilities in Japan indicated that, out of the 114 facilities possessing samples of anthrax or multidrug-resistant TB (or both), 58 did not have manuals on how to handle these dangerous pathogens.[20] And, in China, in the aftermath of SARS, the rush to set up 'Class III pathogen labs' has generated concerns over whether such facilities will have sufficient suitably-trained personnel and meet international biosafety guidelines.[21]

The newest biosafety regulations in East Asia are those of Singapore. In October 2005 the Singapore parliament passed the Biological Agents and Toxins Bill against the backdrop of an increase in the number of Singaporean institutions working with high-risk biological agents. The impetus for extra research on pathogens has been resurgent concern about infectious disease outbreaks of natural origin and the prospect of BW attacks, as well as Singapore's desire to become a centre of biotechnology excellence in Asia. Key provisions for biosafety contained in the new legislation include:

- an operator of a facility handling certain high-risk biological agents is responsible for the safety of staff and visitors to the facility. Risk assessment must be carried out and staff adequately trained.
- the facility and its equipment must be in safe working condition, and biological waste may not be discharged into the environment.
- government approvals for possession and import, and notifications of transfer, are required for high-risk biological agents and toxins to enable effective inventory control and tracking.[22]

In East Asia overall, however, biosafety regulations are lacking. The establishment of more high-containment laboratories in the region would enable a more rapid and effective response to local disease outbreaks – it would, for example, reduce the likelihood of existing WHO influenza laboratories being overwhelmed by requests to analyse samples of H5N1 virus. Nevertheless, the establishment of more laboratories would also potentially increase outbreak risks if they were not managed safely and securely. Of particular concern is a 2006 report on a survey of 300 scientists in 16 Asian countries, commissioned by Sandia National Laboratories in the United States, which showed that pathogen researchers often use insufficient biosafety practices. For example, nearly two-thirds of respondents investigating Japanese encephalitis, avian influenza and SARS – which are all BSL-3 agents – perform their research under BSL-2 conditions.[23] Compounding this problem, it is difficult to know exactly how many putative BSL-3 and BSL-4 laboratories (these are of greatest interest from a security perspective) exist in the region and whether they operate in accordance with international biosafety guidelines. At the Third BWC Review Conference in 1991, the member states agreed to confidence-building measures (CBMs) including exchanges of data on national research centres and BSL-4 laboratories. On the whole, the annual CBM returns of BWC member states have been few in number and of poor quality. The only countries that have recently published their CBM returns on the Internet are Australia, Canada, the United Kingdom and the United States.[24]

Preventing the diversion and misuse of pathogens: biological scientists and biosecurity

Microbiologists and laboratory managers are familiar with the concept of biosafety – it is easy to understand, for example, the importance of protecting oneself from acquiring infections while working on dangerous pathogens. The current emphasis on biosecurity, however, is relatively new. Whereas biosafety focuses on procedures and equipment, biosecurity is more concerned with people's knowledge, choices and behaviour. To explore this notion, the section that follows examines the recent experience of biosecurity regulation and concludes with a discussion of biosecurity in an East Asian context.

'Amerithrax'

In most discussion of biosecurity, the emphasis tends to be on diversion threats posed by outsiders – that is, non-laboratory workers with malign intent who might break into a research facility. This is consistent with the political rhetoric prevalent since 11 September 2001 of 'WMD falling into the hands of terrorists'. It is important, however, not to overlook the threat from insiders – trusted members of staff with access to pathogens and who are familiar with laboratory security procedures and equipment. A rhetorical tag for such a threat might be 'people with WMD deciding to become terrorists'. It is highly likely, for example, that an expert insider with laboratory experience was the perpetrator of the most sophisticated BW attack in history. On 18 September 2001, two letters laced with *B. anthracis* bacteria, addressed to *NBC Nightly News* and the *New York Post*, were postmarked from Trenton, New Jersey. On 3 October, photo editor Robert Stevens was diagnosed with anthrax and placed on a respirator. Two days later, he became the first anthrax death in the United States since 1976. On 9 October, two more anthrax-laced letters, addressed to US Senate Majority Leader Tom Daschle and Senator Patrick Leahy, were again postmarked from Trenton. In the weeks that followed, a total of five Americans died of anthrax and 17 more were infected.[25]

Analyses revealed that the attack spores were examples of the Ames strain of *B. anthracis* – a highly virulent strain originally developed in powder form by the US Army Medical Research Institute for Infectious Diseases (USAMRIID) for testing biological defence systems.[26] Scientists at the Lawrence Livermore National Laboratory used radiocarbon dating to determine that the spores had been cultivated within the previous two years.[27] The anthrax used in the envelope attacks was reportedly 'weapons-grade' – exceptionally free of bacterial residue, of uniform particle size, treated with silica to reduce particle clumping and dispersed easily. Its high concentration (one trillion spores per gram) and purity gave rise to suggestions that the attacks had links to a sophisticated government biodefence programme.[28] The letters inside the envelopes included rhetoric commonly used by Muslim militants. This, and the fact that they were mailed within weeks of the 11 September 2001 attacks on the World Trade Center and the Pentagon, led investigators initially to suppose that Al Qaeda might have been responsible. But the notes also announced the presence of pathogenic bacteria by urging the reader to take antibiotics, which seemed to indicate the perpetrator was more intent on causing panic rather than killing a large number of people. Eventually, Federal Bureau of Investigation (FBI) psychological profilers settled on a 'disaffected American loner' as the most likely perpetrator of the attacks.[29]

Because so much of the circumstantial evidence pointed to a plot hatched and executed within the United States, law-enforcement officials concentrated on biodefence specialists; in particular on scientists familiar with weaponizing pathogens. The FBI investigation focused on army scientists at Fort Detrick – the very ones responsible for protecting the United States from biological attack. In the course of the investigation dubbed 'Amerithrax', US Attorney General John Ashcroft labelled Steven Hatfill a 'person of interest'. Hatfill came under suspicion partly because he formerly worked as a medical researcher at USAMRIID.[30] Despite conducting extensive searches and over 8,000 interviews, the FBI has apparently not gathered sufficient evidence to support charges against Hatfill or anyone else.[31] More than five years later, the case of the anthrax envelopes remains unsolved. The difficulty of bringing the perpetrator to justice underscores the importance of a regime for preventing the diversion and misuse of pathogens in the first place.

Biosecurity regulation in the United States

The story of biosecurity regulation in the United States begins in 1995 when a white supremacist named Larry Wayne Harris ordered three vials of *Y. pestis* bacteria (the causative agent of plague) from the American Type Culture Collection in Virginia. He claimed to be a microbiologist writing a training manual on defence against BW. At the time, the regulation of access to and dissemination of biological agents was almost exclusively about preventing public distribution of unsafe pharmaceutical or other biological products. Thus the only charge on which Harris could be convicted was mail fraud for misusing a laboratory registration number when ordering the plague culture. After this incident, US policy-makers realized it was too easy to obtain pathogenic seed cultures. Under the Antiterrorism and Effective Death Penalty Act 1996, regulations pertaining to the acquisition, transfer, packaging, labelling and handling of 'select' biological agents were tightened to reduce the possibility that such agents could be fraudulently ordered from commercial suppliers.[32] There are currently 82 designated 'select agents' that pose a threat to humans, animals and plants. These are divided into three categories (A, B and C) based on assessments of ease of dissemination or transmission, mortality and public health impact, ability to cause panic and social disruption, and special requirements for public health preparedness.[33] Federal regulations require any laboratory that possesses one or more of these agents to enforce and adhere to specific security measures. These include: facility registration and designation of a responsible official; risk assessments for individuals with access to listed agents; biosecurity plans; agent transfer rules; safety and security training and inspections; notification after theft, loss or release of a listed agent; and record maintenance.[34]

In the aftermath of the World Trade Center disaster and the anthrax envelope attacks, the US Congress passed the Uniting and Strengthening America by Providing Appropriate Tools Required to Intercept and Obstruct Terrorism (USA PATRIOT) Act 2001. This legislation sets requirements for the appropriate use of select biological agents, specifies people who should be restricted from working with them, and imposes criminal and civil penalties for inappropriate use. The Public Health Security and Bioterrorism Preparedness Act 2002 requires authorities at research and medical facilities to report work with select agents, and to submit the names of employees with a legitimate need for access to pathogens to the Health and Human Services Secretary and the Attorney General. These names are checked against criminal, immigration and national security databases for possible 'restricted person' status.[35]

An important lesson from the US experience is that biosecurity regulation must strike a balance between maximizing security benefits while doing the least amount of harm to legitimate research. The biotechnology sector is simultaneously a potential locus of disease-based security threats and a crucial ally for governments seeking to resist such threats. The sector performs basic research on pathogenic micro-organisms, produces vaccines and other drugs, and instructs health professionals on how to use them. Too much biosecurity might cripple commercial and academic enterprise in the biological sciences and thereby diminish the ability of the public health system – particularly its diagnostic and patient-care elements – to respond to an outbreak event.

Many US scientists have decided to discontinue or not pursue research on regulated agents, rather than bear the associated financial and administrative burdens. Scientists at Stanford University, for example, destroyed or transferred collections of *F. tularensis* and *Y. pestis* because they believed the burdens of the select agent regulations outweighed the scientific need to maintain stocks on campus.[36] An additional concern, exacerbated by the recent prosecution of plague expert Thomas Butler, is that fear of personal legal trouble might also induce some individuals to turn away from research on particular infectious diseases.

The plague and Thomas Butler

Biological scientists around the world would have been disturbed by the sight of 62-year-old Thomas Butler, a well-known plague researcher, in prison garb with his hands bound. In 2003, the former chief of the infectious diseases division at Texas Tech University was the first US scientist to be tried on biosecurity-related charges. Butler faced a 69-count federal indictment, including charges that he smuggled plague bacteria and lied to the FBI. Here was a scientist with the ability and intention to increase his country's security against infectious disease threats who ran foul of laws designed to do likewise.

The story of Thomas Butler's encounter with US biosecurity regulations begins in the mid-1990s at a time when US policy-makers were beginning to contemplate more seriously the prospect of biological attacks perpetrated by non-state actors. Plague was a particularly hot topic – the defector Ken Alibek, a former Soviet BW researcher, had revealed that his country had mass-produced *Y. pestis*, and concerns deepened further in 1995 when the US government arrested Larry Wayne Harris for ordering plague samples under false pretences. Butler, as the author of over 30 peer-reviewed articles, reviews and chapters on plague, was in a good position to undertake research that might address some of his government's concerns. His most recent project was spurred by his realization that the antibiotics most commonly recommended to treat plague were outdated, had problems with bacterial resistance and/or were not ordinarily stocked in American pharmacies. He believed it was important to obtain clinical data to show that more modern and widely available antibiotics could also effectively treat patients suffering from plague. There would have been ethical prohibitions against testing antibiotics on humans intentionally infected with plague for research purposes, so Butler had to go where a natural outbreak was occurring. In 2000 he began a collaborative project with colleagues at the University of Tanzania to study the efficacy of gentamicin and doxycycline therapy in plague patients.[37] In the mountains of north-eastern Tanzania, where plague is endemic, Butler and his collaborators drew fluid samples from the 'buboes' (swollen lymph nodes) of patients to confirm the presence of *Y. pestis*.[38]

In April 2002, Butler packed his fluid samples in dry ice and placed them in his footlocker for the flight home to the US via London. The practice of researchers carrying infectious disease samples packed in metal boxes on commercial flights had been common for decades.[39] In London, a fellow microbiologist gave Butler fresh dry ice to keep his samples cold. The next day, Butler travelled into Texas and back to his university laboratory. On 23 June, he drove 1,200 kilometres to the US Centers for Disease Control and Prevention (CDC) laboratory at Fort Collins, Colorado. The plague researchers at CDC had already agreed to test Butler's Tanzanian samples in their laboratory, which at that stage was the only one in the United States certified to do so. On 9 September he sent plague samples back to Tanzania via FedEx, a commercial courier. On 1 October, Butler flew to Washington, DC, thence travelled to USAMRIID in Maryland with a third set of samples – the USAMRIID researchers were keen to add Tanzanian strains of plague to their reference collections.[40] From a public health perspective, Butler's research was a resounding success and his team submitted a manuscript to the prestigious medical journal, *The Lancet*. Their work in Tanzania had showed that the antibiotics doxycycline and gentamicin, readily available in the United States, were effective in treating plague.[41] From a legal perspective, however, the crucial point was that Butler had conveyed his plague samples without the necessary authorization and permits. This omission was exposed in the course of an investigation into an incident at his own laboratory.

On 13 January 2003, Butler reported to Texas Tech University administrators that 30 vials of *Y. pestis* brought back from Tanzania had gone missing. He said at the time that he presumed they had been stolen from his laboratory. Concerned about the possibility of deliberate pathogen misuse, university officials decided to contact law-enforcement authorities. The FBI and other agencies sent 60 investigators to scour the university and the town of Lubbock (population 200,000) in search of the missing vials, and Lubbock-area hospitals and medical personnel were notified to be on the look-out for cases of plague. After interrogation during which he waived his right to a lawyer, Butler signed a statement that he had accidentally destroyed the vials of *Y. pestis* and had declared them missing 'to demonstrate why [he] could not account for the plague bacteria that had been in [his] possession'. The FBI then arrested him on 16 January for allegedly lying to its agents. Butler later said he had signed under duress, pressured by the FBI to allay public fears about any dangers.[42] Texas Tech University banned Butler from his laboratory and began the process of firing him. The investigation of Butler and his recent activities on the Tanzanian project revealed that he had possibly violated federal laws when he failed to report properly that he was carrying specimens of *Y. pestis* (a select agent). In April 2003, a federal grand jury indicted Butler on 15 counts including smuggling, lying to investigators and illegal transportation of hazardous biological materials. In addition, he was to be tried on charges of fraud and embezzlement, but these were in no way related to the original disappearance of vials that first attracted the involvement of law-enforcement officials. They arose out of contractual disputes Butler had with his university in connection with research he conducted for two pharmaceutical companies. Such disputes are normally handled through civil, not criminal, proceedings.[43]

At no point was Butler accused of being, or seeking to aid, a 'terrorist'. Butler's lawyers argued that the expanded charges were 'a face-saving attempt by the government to secure a conviction at any cost'; a scheme to hide the fact that the 'bioterrorism' scare ignited by the FBI's initial search of Texas Tech University was unjustified.[44] Many scientists agreed that the US government had gone too far; that it was prosecuting Butler in a manner grossly disproportionate to the offences alleged. Supporters of Butler suggested that the original confusion over the missing plague bacteria was the result of mere absent-mindedness on the part of a scientist who had always been lax about paperwork. It has apparently long been common practice for scientists to transport specimens personally, a habit referred to as 'VIP' for 'vials in pocket'.[45] The US government maintained, however, that Butler's actions represented 'perilous naivety and sloppiness' in adhering to restrictions on the handling of hazardous pathogens.[46] An editorial in the *Washington Post* echoed this sentiment, arguing that tighter enforcement of the legal rules about handling disease agents is not unreasonable in a world in which 'bioterrorism' poses a real threat: 'In post-Sept. 11 America, the government would be derelict if it did not insist on knowing who has what bugs.'[47]

In December 2003, a Texas jury found Butler guilty of multiple counts of embezzlement and fraud but acquitted him of lying to the FBI about the theft of *Y. pestis* vials from his laboratory. On the charges involving smuggling and mishandling of plague samples, he was acquitted of smuggling samples into the United States from Tanzania and illegally taking them to government laboratories in Colorado and Maryland. But his exoneration was not complete – Butler was found guilty on three charges related to the shipment of samples to a Tanzanian researcher without the proper permit, the package having been labelled merely as 'laboratory materials'.[48] On 10 March 2004 he was sentenced to two years in prison. The judge had cut seven years off a possible standard nine-year sentence set by federal guidelines, citing testimony that the bacteria shipment was done for humanitarian reasons and that the US Department of Commerce would have approved a transportation permit had Butler applied for one. The judge also cited Butler's early work on treatment of diarrhoeal diseases and oral rehydration as having 'led to the salvage of millions of lives throughout the world'.[49]

Thomas Butler was a scientist caught in a clash between longstanding scientific practices and new biosecurity regulations. The circumstances surrounding his arrest, trial and sentencing indicate that he was both an asset and a liability to the United States in its quest to avert infectious disease threats. Butler's research on possible new plague treatments was clearly considered highly valuable for the purposes of US domestic security – the CDC, USAMRIID and the Food and Drug Administration (FDA) had all wanted to work with Butler on biodefence initiatives.[50] In an article in *Clinical Infectious Diseases*, 14 of Butler's colleagues stated: 'we think it makes very little sense to have removed from action such a knowledgeable and active clinician and clinical investigator who was working to protect us from plague – such removal is akin to shooting ourselves in the foot.'[51] If the US government was seeking to make an example of Butler in order to scare scientists into obeying strict new biosecurity laws, it was a risky tactic. Some scientists have predicted that, to the contrary, the Butler case will drive researchers away from collaborations with government on biodefence and thus undermine national security.[52] In August 2003, the presidents of the NAS and the US Institute of Medicine protested about the treatment of Butler by federal prosecutors, taking the rare step of writing to Attorney General John Ashcroft. The letter voiced their concern that the prosecution might cause other scientists to be 'discouraged from embarking upon or continuing crucial bioterrorism-related scientific research – thereby adversely affecting the nation's ability to fully utilize such research capabilities in preparing defenses against possible bioterrorist attacks.'[53] In essence, this was a warning about the security pitfalls of overzealous law enforcement.

Ironically, from a security perspective, the biggest mystery of the Butler case remains unsolved. Butler said that the 30 vials of *Y. pestis* went missing from his laboratory; he did not destroy them. The trial jury believed him and so, presumably, a quantity of plague pathogen remains unaccounted for.

Biosecurity, the BWC and East Asia

In the United States, regulators are gradually acknowledging the wisdom of accommodating scientists' concerns in order to make the evolving biosecurity regime effective. However, some US scholars and policy-makers are concerned that biosecurity is only truly effective if implemented on a global scale.[54] To achieve this, the task of balancing competing interests is likely to be even more difficult than at the domestic level. It is highly unlikely that the US model of biosecurity regulation could be directly applied elsewhere – specific biosecurity measures cannot be instituted on a 'one size fits all' basis. For example, few countries would have sufficient bureaucratic and law-enforcement infrastructures to support the extensive criminal background checks carried out by US agencies. Other countries with smaller (or non-existent) biotechnology sectors might deem biosecurity measures unnecessary. And, in the developing world especially, some countries may be so preoccupied with addressing naturally occurring infectious disease threats that preventing deliberate disease seems a secondary concern.

The diversity of interests, priorities and concerns among countries facing infectious disease threats means the United States would need to be flexible in its call for worldwide biosecurity. Other members of the international community would need to be persuaded that biosecurity is justified for reasons beyond assuaging self-interested US concerns about 'bioterrorism' – most compelling would be an argument that adhering to a global biosecurity regime would benefit global public health. As no other country fears the public health consequences of non-state BW use to the same extent as the United States, it may need to provide incentives to countries unable or unwilling to invest in biosecurity. Developing nations might, for example, be willing to implement biosecurity standards in exchange for financial and technical assistance in the struggle against ongoing infectious disease threats such as HIV/AIDS, malaria and TB.[55]

It is important to acknowledge, however, that the establishment of a global biosecurity regime would not simply be about the security interests of the United States. The BWC in effect already requires that such a regime be created by the combined national efforts of all its member states. To comply with Article IV of the Convention, it is not enough that a state itself does not develop, produce, stockpile or otherwise acquire, retain or transfer biological weapons. Rather, as stated in the Final Declaration of the 1996 Fourth BWC Review Conference, member states need to 'ensure, through the review and/or adoption of national measures, the effective fulfilment of their obligations under the Convention in order, *inter alia*, to exclude use of biological and toxin weapons in terrorist or criminal activity'.[56] This section assesses the extent to which biosecurity is being addressed by the countries of East Asia. In November 2003, the BWC member states met in Geneva to 'discuss, and promote common understanding and effective action' on

1   national measures to implement the Convention, including penal legislation and
2   national mechanisms for security and oversight of pathogenic microorganisms and toxins.[57]

Although the meeting had no mandate to make decisions, the member states 'agreed on the value' of:

* enacting, reviewing or updating national laws for implementing the prohibitions of the BWC, and for enhancing the security of pathogens;
* cooperation between member states with differing legal and constitutional arrangements, and the provision of legal and technical assistance to those states needing to frame or expand their legislation; and
* comprehensive national measures to secure pathogen collections and ensure such materials are not accessible to persons who might misuse them.[58]

Most governments in East Asia have yet to apply much effort to enhancing biosecurity beyond simple criminalization. For example, the Malaysian Penal

Code criminalizes malignant acts 'likely to spread the infection of any disease dangerous to life', and the legislation defines a 'terrorist act' to include an act that involves the use of any microbial or biological agent or toxin.[59] Similarly, the Criminal Law of the People's Republic of China prescribes criminal penalties for 'any illegal manufacturing, trading in, transporting, storing, using, stealing, snatching or robbing' of infectious pathogens.[60] However, criminalizing the diversion and misuse of pathogens is no substitute for establishing legally binding biosecurity measures aimed at preventing such occurrences. In contemplating biosecurity regulation, governments in East Asia will likely seek to balance possible security risks against the need to encourage and retain biological scientists. At present, weak or non-existent oversight of pathogen research may in fact be an incentive to work in East Asia and a key factor in supporting the regional economy's biotechnology sector.

Among the countries of East Asia, the leader on biosecurity is Japan. Formerly, the Japanese government provided private sector entities, including research institutes, universities, manufacturers and academic or business associations, with guidelines on desirable biosecurity measures. It was up to those entities to institute such measures voluntarily and to self-regulate their activities. In the aftermath of the 2001 anthrax attacks in the United States, Japan ramped up the level of government oversight. In particular, its Basic Policy on Responding to Biological and Chemical Terrorism now includes enhanced management of pathogens of potential BW concern.[61] At the 2003 Meeting of BWC Member States, Japan contributed a paper on measures for strengthening biosecurity which recommended: lists of dangerous pathogens and toxins; monitoring of facilities and individuals that handle controlled pathogens and toxins; monitoring the transfer of controlled pathogens; and physical security measures applied to laboratories and other facilities handling controlled pathogens and toxins.[62] It remains to be seen, however, whether other countries in East Asia will pursue biosecurity with equal vigour as a matter of national importance.

Experiments, security and codes of conduct

In addition to finding physical and procedural solutions, biosecurity is about individual scientists conducting their research with a security consciousness. Determining the appropriate nature and extent of risk management is a vexed issue because the scientific and national-security communities have different objectives, cultures and norms. As a consequence, they are likely to weigh the costs and benefits of proposed policy measures differently. According to a long-standing 'empiricist' conception of science that lasted until about the 1960s, it was widely assumed that the purpose of scientific inquiry was to produce an objective account of a natural world that existed independently of the inquiry. An important implication of the empiricist conception is that what scientists do in their laboratories does not engage moral or political issues. This view has since been moderated by powerful critiques arguing that the laboratory walls do not and should not symbolize a scientist's splendid isolation. Rather, his or her production of knowledge is subject to social and cultural influences. Nevertheless, empiricist notions – the social isolation of scientists, the objectivity of science, and the linearity of scientific progress – remain a powerful subtext in most forms of scientific education.[63]

On the issue of scientists' security consciousness, it is useful at the outset to compare microbiologists with nuclear physicists. In the second half of the twentieth century, an intellectual infrastructure evolved with respect to nuclear weapons that provided a common framework for understanding between nuclear physicists and security analysts. Since the invention of the atomic bomb, nuclear physicists have moved between universities, national weapons laboratories and government policy offices. Most are accustomed to dealing with the burdens of security clearances, protecting sensitive information and having research results kept secret. No such infrastructure exists for understanding the security challenges posed by biotechnology. Historically, security analysts and biological scientists have not had enough interaction to have necessitated the development of a common 'language'.[64] The two branches of science also differ in scale and location. During the Cold War, data on nuclear weapons was held closely by only a small cadre of nuclear physicists. By contrast, the American Society of Microbiology alone has 42,000 members, with almost one-third of them from outside the United States.[65] And unlike the historical domination of aspects of nuclear physics by military programmes, modern advances in biotechnology are today being driven largely by academic and commercial research.

Moving beyond adherence to legally enforceable biosecurity regulations, this section explores the security consciousness of biological scientists in two important dimensions. The first is the issue of so-called 'experiments of concern' and the security implications of research that produces dangerous pathogens through genetic modification. The second dimension involves codes of conduct for scientists, which encompasses issues such as: the reliability of self-regulation by scientists; policies on what research findings ought not to be published in scientific journals; and whether there should be a separate code of conduct for defence scientists.

Experiments of concern

According to a 2004 NAS report, 'experiments of concern' are those that would:

1   demonstrate how to render a vaccine ineffective;
2   confer resistance to therapeutically useful antibiotics or antiviral agents;
3   enhance the virulence of a pathogen or render a non-pathogen virulent;
4   increase the transmissibility of a pathogen;
5   alter the host range of a pathogen;

6   enable the evasion of diagnosis and/or detection by established methods; or

7   enable the weaponization of a biological agent or toxin.[66]

To this list might be added:

8   genetic sequencing of a pathogen; and
9   synthesizing the genome of a pathogen.

As set out in Table 8.2, there is a 'dual-use' dilemma associated with each type of experiment – that is, the results could be applied for both benign and malevolent purposes.

Of particular security significance were the unintended consequences of research by a group of Australian scientists, published by the *Journal of Virology* in 2001, who were attempting to produce an infectious contraceptive for mice, which periodically breed out of control in parts of Australia. The scientists spliced a single foreign gene into a mild mousepox virus in the hope of creating a genetically engineered sterility treatment – the gene, interleukin-4 (IL-4), helps to regulate immune system reactions. The effect, however, was to create not a contraceptive but a strain of mousepox so powerful that it killed even those mice inoculated against the virus.[67] A disturbing implication of this result is that adding an IL-4 gene might similarly increase the fatality rate of smallpox (or some other poxvirus that infects humans) and potentially allow the virus to overcome vaccination.

Scientists on another project, carried out partly to draw attention to BW threats, spent three years synthesizing DNA corresponding to the 7,500 chemical units of poliomyelitis (polio) virus. When the assembled virus was injected into mice, they were paralysed and killed.[68] The polio project proved that eradicating a virus in the wild might not mean it is gone forever – conceivably, scientists may soon be able to apply the same technique to synthesize more complex viruses such as Ebola using blueprints available in scientific archives and from biological supplies purchased through the mail. The mousepox and polio experiments, and the publicity they received, thus sensitized politicians and security analysts to the need to raise awareness among scientists about the security implications of particular research.

Notwithstanding such concerns, the genetic engineering of viruses can have a broader public health purpose against which security considerations might not weigh as heavily. For example, the WHO is presently sponsoring research to find out whether H5N1 avian influenza could trigger a human pandemic. The hope is that, by 'reassorting' (mixing) H5N1 with human influenza viruses in the laboratory, scientists may determine how dangerous the hybrid virus would be and the likelihood of it causing a pandemic. Such experiments could help to determine whether there is some natural barrier to the reassortment of H5N1 or whether the world has simply been lucky. They are controversial, however, because they could create dangerous new viruses

Table 8.2 Dual-use dilemmas

Experiment	Dual-use dilemma
Rendering a vaccine ineffective	1 It is important to know whether or how vaccines can be made ineffective, to enable their improvement or identification of alternative treatments. 2 Rendering a vaccine ineffective could allow the deployment of BW that cannot be resisted using standard vaccination techniques.
Conferring resistance to therapeutically useful antibiotics or antiviral agents	1 Conferring antibiotic resistance may provide data that helps to improve the administration of antibiotics, or it could be used to test the efficacy of alternative antibiotics. 2 The same technique could also be used to produce BW agents that are resistant to common antibiotics.
Enhancing the virulence of a pathogen or rendering a non-pathogen virulent	1 For public health reasons, it may be important to know whether or how the virulence of a pathogen that exists in nature can increase. 2 An 'enhanced' pathogen, if deployed in a biological attack, would inflict more human damage than normal.
Increasing the transmissibility of a pathogen	1 For treatment and public health planning purposes, it may be important to know whether a naturally-occurring infectious disease threat could be worsened by the evolution of a pathogen into a more transmissible form. 2 A pathogen might be more useful for BW purposes if it is more easily transmitted through a population.
Altering the host range of a pathogen	1 It may be important to know whether a non-zoonotic disease can become, or is close to becoming, a zoonotic agent. 2 The use in a biological attack of an animal disease agent that has been engineered to infect humans would be devastating because people would have no immunity to the disease.

Enabling the evasion of diagnosis and/or detection by established methods	1 It may be important to know whether a pathogen has the potential to mutate naturally into an undetectable form so that new diagnostic and detection techniques may be devised. 2 Pathogens engineered to evade diagnosis and/or detection would be well-suited for a covert BW attack, and the delay in diagnosis and subsequent treatment would increase the resulting human damage.
Enabling the weaponization of a biological agent or toxin	1 Understanding weaponization processes may facilitate the development of protections against a potential BW incident. 2 Weaponization for 'threat-assessment' purposes is likely to be interpreted by outsiders as the production of BW, thus endangering the norm against their use, making biological attacks more likely.
Genetic sequencing of a pathogen	1 Sequencing the genetic code of entire pathogens or specific genes of pathogens could assist in understanding the nature of the pathogen and in the development of new vaccines or treatments for the disease it causes. 2 Gene sequence data could be used to reconstruct a pathogen (or one with its harmful characteristics) for deployment against a target population with no natural immunity
Synthesizing the genome of a pathogen	1 Synthesis of the genomes of viruses theoretically allows the introduction of mutations or novel sequences that can be used to study the function of particular genes or regulatory sequences. 2 Synthesis technology would obviate the need to source pathogens from natural reservoirs in other parts of the world or from other laboratories. It can facilitate reconstruction of extinct pathogens and could enable construction of novel pathogens.

that would need to be destroyed or kept extremely secure. And, after the three SARS accidents in East Asia, biosafety concerns compound the controversy over whether H5N1 experiments are wise.

Codes of conduct

The potentially grave security implications of 'experiments of concern' highlight the powerful position held by scientists with access to pathogens and knowledge of what makes them dangerous. For the most part, such scientists are conscientiously determined to use their position for the good of humankind. The possibility remains, however, that scientific skills and knowledge might be applied in a manner hostile or recklessly indifferent to human life. The imposition of legal rules, often resisted by scientists, can go only so far in addressing that risk. A complementary approach to avoiding non-peaceful applications of biotechnology is through ethical norms agreed to by scientists themselves. In 2005, the BWC member states had a mandate to discuss and promote effective action on the content, promulgation and adoption of codes of conduct for scientists. At a Meeting of Experts in June of that year, China, Indonesia, Japan and South Korea reported the existence of ethical guidelines for scientists in each country, although none were specifically couched in terms of addressing BW-related risks. However, the idea of codes of conduct as a security device is new to much of the world – governments and scientists in East Asia are not alone in lacking established ethical guidelines for pathogen research.

Regarding the nature and content of codes of conduct, it is generally agreed that governments cannot simply impose codes of conduct upon scientists. Rather, a bottom-up approach in which scientists adhere to codes voluntarily is an essential part of monitoring the security significance of research in the biological sciences. Researchers naturally abhor restraints, but the degree to which they accept them depends upon how well they understand the legitimacy of such restraints. In terms of expertise, biological scientists are in a good position to recognize the potential misuses of their work, and to decide the ways in which biological science might be most efficiently governed. And, at a practical level, local oversight of scientists may be more effective than national oversight because researchers are arguably more readily influenced by peers within their own immediate research environment. However, biological scientists are not the only community of interest as regards the security implications of their work – others include, for example, lawyers, doctors, policy-makers and BWC specialists – and thus it would be inappropriate to characterize codes of conduct as the concern of scientists alone. Rather, such codes should combine both top-down and bottom-up elements, with the conduct of scientists receiving multidisciplinary scrutiny as to its security significance.

A working paper prepared by Australia for the June 2005 BWC Meeting of Experts in Geneva contained a suggestion that there be three layers of codes of conduct:

1　a *universal code* containing guiding principles – a short, aspirational code containing general principles and referring to ethical norms, to be implemented using a top-down approach.
2　*codes of ethics* developed by scientific societies – these could be new codes, or elements could be added to existing societal codes. Elements could include general principles, and awareness-raising about dual-use dilemmas in the biological sciences and about BWC obligations.
3　*codes of practice* (institutional or workplace codes) – these could be new codes or elements could be added to existing workplace codes. Elements could include: full awareness by the scientific community of national laws pertaining to biological science activities and of the need to comply with such laws, and awareness-raising about ethical considerations including scientific responsibility when working on certain research projects that may lead to discoveries that make BW more effective.[69]

In deciding on particular points of ethical guidance, the challenge is to have codes of conduct that are specific enough to have a positive effect and sufficiently flexible to accommodate technological change. The minimum and primary purpose of a code would be to raise awareness among scientists and others about the possible misuse of pathogens. Beyond that, a governance regime could include one or more of four elements:

1　*opacity* – should there be restrictions on publication or other dissemination of certain types of research because of their potential for abuse?
2　*transparency* – are particular types of research and experimentation so sensitive regarding their potential BW application that they merit extraordinary obligations for openness?
3　*responsibility* – what is the obligation of research scientists to call attention to or clarify the activities of colleagues that may appear suspicious?
4　*constraint* – beyond biosafety considerations, are there areas of research or types of experiments that are so dangerous, or so explicitly linked to offensive BW activity, that they should not be conducted at all?[70]

The NAS report of 2004 sought to make recommendations that achieved an appropriate balance between the pursuit of national security and scientific advances to improve human health and welfare. It proposed a system that combined voluntary self-governance by the scientific community and expansion of the existing regulatory process that had grown out of concerns in the 1970s about genetically modified organisms. Key recommendations were:

1　that national and international professional societies and related organizations and institutions create programmes to educate scientists about the nature of the dual-use dilemma in biotechnology and their responsibilities to mitigate its risks;

2   that the US government create a review system for seven classes of 'experiments of concern';
3   that there be self-governance by scientists and scientific journals to review publications for their potential national security risks; and
4   that a National Science Advisory Board for Biodefense be created to provide advice, guidance, and leadership for the proposed system of review and oversight.[71]

Following the recommendations of the NAS report, in March 2004 the US government announced plans to establish a 25-member National Science Advisory Board for Biosecurity (NSABB). The role of the NSABB is to establish guidelines for the security review of sensitive biological research projects in academia and, on a voluntary basis, in the private sector. Its mandate does not extend, however, to the review of classified biodefence research initiated and funded by the US government and conducted at federal facilities.[72] Although the approach of relying mainly on self-governance is likely to receive more support from scientists than a set of rules imposed from the top down, the NAS recommendations may be criticized on at least two grounds. One criticism is that, because research in the biological sciences is essentially an international endeavour, national structures for oversight do not go far enough. Accordingly, an international organization, possibly along the lines of the WHO Variola Advisory Committee, which oversees US and Russian work on smallpox, might need to be established to monitor and review other research. Second, contrary to NAS expectations, recent experience suggests that review of research findings by journal editors at the publication stage might not amount to much of a 'filter' at all.

The publication dilemma

A 2002 article in *BioScience* entitled 'Biological warfare targeted at livestock' featured an editor's note that portions of the article were 'intentionally left vague to prevent misuse'.[73] This reflects a fear that would-be BW perpetrators might acquire a deadly capability just by reading the open scientific literature. In February 2003, in response to security concerns of this kind, a group of 32 journal editors and authors published a 'Statement on the consideration of biodefence and biosecurity' in *Nature*. The statement acknowledged that 'there is information that, although we cannot now capture it with lists of definitions, presents enough risk of use by terrorists that it should not be published'. At the same time, it was considered vital to 'protect the integrity of the scientific process by publishing manuscripts of high quality, in sufficient detail to permit reproducibility'. The rationale for this was couched in both scientific and security terms – without the independent verification required for scientific progress, the statement explained, 'we can neither advance biomedical research nor provide the knowledge base for building strong biodefence systems'. The authors announced that they would therefore weigh the potential harm of publication against the scientific benefits of a submitted research article, and make the decision to modify or publish manuscripts on that basis.[74]

As an illustration of this process, in October 2005 *Science* published research findings on the traits that made the 'Spanish' influenza virus so virulent. Using the recently completed genetic code sequence of the 1918 H1N1 virus (obtained from the preserved tissue of a 1918 victim), the researchers used reverse genetics to generate a virus identical to that which caused the pandemic.[75] The authors and the journal editors acknowledged that this information, once published, could potentially be used by someone wishing to reconstruct the 1918 influenza virus for a malign purpose. However, a last-minute review by the NSABB concluded that the scientific benefit of the future use of this information far outweighed the potential risk of misuse.[76] And a covering editorial in *Science* emphasized the 'good news' that this latest information on the 1918 influenza virus could facilitate 'the development of new therapies and vaccines to protect against another such pandemic'.[77]

From a purely scientific perspective, a culture of openness and free exchange of ideas allows researchers to build on the results of others. It also exposes scientific results to critical scrutiny so that mistakes can be recognized and corrected sooner rather than later. If the assumptions and methods underlying an experiment are not tested for their soundness, research that follows on from it might be flawed. In the area of therapeutic research on pathogens, another reason for openness might be that medicine is based on universal humanitarian principles that stand above the self-interest of individual nations. There is also the argument, advanced on public health grounds, that people deserve clear and accurate information on infectious disease risks and their protective options. Despite the numerous arguments in favour of openness, however, it is not the case that scientists have an unfettered freedom to research any topic and to publish the results. Restrictions on publication have long been a fact of life for scientists working in security-sensitive areas, such as weapons-related nuclear research. Now, as a consequence of advances in biotechnology, microbiologists too are increasingly required to consider security when contemplating publication. There are clearly cases where outright censorship would be appropriate – for example, an article describing how to synthesize the smallpox virus or how to weaponize anthrax bacteria. However, a recent test case shows how the 'filter' of review by journal editors allowed publication of research findings showing how to cause a large-scale outbreak of botulism.

In May 2005, the US Department of Health and Human Services (DHHS) made an unprecedented request to *Proceedings of the National Academy of Sciences* (*PNAS*) to withdraw a paper that the journal had planned to publish online on 30 May 2005. The paper modelled an attack involving the deliberate contamination of the US milk supply with botulinum toxin. It estimated the extent of illness and death that would result and spelled out what steps the government and industry could take to prevent such an attack.[78] While the *PNAS* editors deliberated on whether to proceed with publication, one of the paper's authors (Lawrence Wein) published an opinion piece in the *New York Times* that described the study in some detail.[79] On 28 June, *PNAS* posted the toxin paper in full on its website in advance of print publication the following month.[80] In a covering editorial, NAS president Bruce Alberts explained that publication was justified because '[a]ll of the critical information in this article that could be useful to a terrorist ... [is] immediately accessible on the World Wide Web through a simple Google search'.[81]

The botulinum toxin article was a test case for balancing scientific freedom and national security, and one that highlighted a clash of cultures. Wein, a professor of management at Stanford University, sought to publish the paper in order to 'nudge' US policy-makers into better protecting the nation's milk supply.[82] In its letter to *PNAS*, however, the DHHS said the paper 'is a road map for terrorists and publication is not in the interests of the United States'.[83] It is too early to judge the security implications of the *PNAS* decision, although permitting publication because information is already available on the Internet is a dubious justification. Even through 'a simple Google search', it takes considerable time and research skills to assemble data from various sources and transform it into an integrated and clearly explained whole. Arguably, someone planning to contaminate the US milk supply has now been spared a lot of bother. Another lesson to be derived from the case of the 'toxic milk' article is that journal publication is by no means the only avenue for exposing research findings. If authors disagreed with an editor's decision to censor, they could simply apply for publication in another journal. Moreover, research findings are often presented first at meetings and conferences, and via email and telephone, and it is becoming increasingly common for researchers to post interim results on websites.

Concerns about publication appear to be driven primarily by the view that pathogen misuse would be something perpetrated by someone who is *not* already a skilled scientist. For example, in September 2003 the editor of *Science*, Donald Kennedy, commented that the scientific community was under increasing pressure from the US government to reduce the chances that one of its articles would 'end up in a cave in Afghanistan with yellow highlighter all over it'.[84] A contrasting view is that would-be perpetrators of biological attacks might not need to rely upon newly published research results. The most sophisticated biological attack by a non-state actor has been that which used weaponized anthrax bacteria in 2001, yet nobody has ever published a paper on how to weaponize anthrax. As discussed previously, the attack was probably the action of one or more scientists from inside the US defence establishment.

A code of conduct for defence scientists

Wherever a proposed code of conduct goes beyond broad, exhortative statements about avoiding malign applications of biotechnology, it is likely to generate controversy. This is clearly the case in areas such as research oversight and publication policies. However, the issue likely to pose the greatest challenges is the need for ethical conduct within national 'defensive' BW programmes. Arguably, among the thousands of scientists working with dangerous pathogens, most in need of ethical guidance are those who work at the fringes of what is permissible under the BWC. A special code of conduct for defence scientists would be an ongoing supplement to any background checks and psychological tests that precede commencement of work.

The former USAMRIID scientist Steven Hatfill attracted attention in the 'Amerithrax' investigation because the FBI were looking for people able to carry out biological attacks. By the time the Iraq War started in 2003, however, Hatfill had also attracted the attention of the US Department of Defense. Months after he came under FBI scrutiny and lost his government security clearance, Hatfill was engaged by the DIA to train an elite team on ways to search for BW.[85] That two different parts of the US government would be interested in Hatfill demonstrates how he was simultaneously regarded in BW terms as both a defender and a potential perpetrator. Although Hatfill has not been convicted of or charged with involvement in the 2001 anthrax attacks, his designation by the FBI as a 'person of interest' supports the proposition that personnel inside a biodefence facility are a potentially serious avenue for pathogen diversion.

The kind of research that comes closest to crossing the line between permitted defensive and illegal offensive work is that which is undertaken for 'threat-assessment' purposes. This involves exploring the offensive applications of biological agents in order to develop appropriate countermeasures. From a security perspective, this gives rise to two challenges. First, scientists who conduct experiments on the offensive side of BW have knowledge of techniques and access to materials which, in the event of a change of mind and an opportunity presenting itself, they could use for malign purposes. Second, beyond risks to domestic biosecurity, threat-assessment projects carry international security significance if they undermine the BWC. In November 2002 a group of non-government organizations (NGOs) drafted recommendations for a code of conduct for biodefence programmes and distributed them to country delegations attending the resumed session of the Fifth BWC Review Conference in Geneva. Of particular relevance to BW threat-assessment projects, the draft code included the following statements:

> The Convention's stated goal is to preclude the use of biological weapons under any circumstances; therefore it is not permissible, even for defensive purposes, to construct delivery mechanisms designed for

(i.e., having a design that is appropriate for) hostile use, whether or not hostile use is intended at the time of construction.

Construction of novel (i.e., not previously-existing) biological agents (including single gene changes) for threat assessment is incompatible with the spirit and intent of the Convention, and should be disavowed.

Aerosolization or other dissemination of active biological agents should be performed only in fully-contained bench-scale environments and only for the purposes of detection, prophylaxis or medical treatment.[86]

Conclusion

In East Asia, the number of people and laboratories devoted to research on pathogenic micro-organisms is increasing for at least three reasons: its commercial potential; a perceived need to develop drugs to counter state or non-state use of BW; and post-SARS concerns about outbreak events of natural origin. As more laboratories and scientists are assigned to address the region's infectious disease problems, it is vital that such research does not increase the risk of outbreak events resulting from accidents or the deliberate misuse of a pathogen. Three recent incidents of laboratory workers being exposed to the SARS virus have highlighted the necessity for safe research practices. Although some countries already have comprehensive biosafety regimes in place, biosafety regulation in the region as a whole is insufficient. Biosecurity regulation in the region also lags dangerously behind expansions in the biotechnology industry, although the solution is not for every country in East Asia to replicate the expensive and complex biosecurity measures evolving in the United States. An important lesson from the US experience is that a degree of flexibility is required to enable the scientific advances and industrial developments necessary to resist infectious disease threats – if regulation is too onerous, many scientists will simply opt out of potentially life-saving pathogen research.

The security consciousness of biological scientists might, in some cases, lead to decisions that some research simply should not be carried out at all. However, the problem lies in obtaining agreement among scientists and among the various other communities of interest on exactly when the security risks of particular research outweigh the public health benefits. Codes of conduct are one possible means of addressing the risk that scientists might deliberately or inadvertently contribute to the malign misuse of pathogens. Such codes would be most effective if they were adopted using a combined top-down and bottom-up approach. Governments cannot imbue scientists with security concerns if they are not convinced such concerns are legitimate; however, scientists are not the only community of interest as regards the implications of their work. A precedent for scientific self-governance exists in the process that has guided recombinant DNA research since the 1970s. The revision of research findings by journal editors is another possible means of discouraging contentious experiments and studies, although recent experience suggests that individual editors may feel unable or unwilling to prevent the dissemination of information.

The area of pathogen research that most requires ethical guidance is work conducted inside ostensibly defensive BW programmes. It is necessary, first, to ensure that scientists skilled and knowledgeable in the area of biological warfare do not abuse their position. Second, the line of legality between offensive and defensive applications of biological agents, although it can be difficult to discern, must be policed rigorously. From an international security perspective, the greatest risk of crossing that line is posed by investigations into the offensive applications of pathogens for threat-assessment purposes. For the purpose of bolstering the norm against BW, regulating the conduct of defence scientists is critical because these are the scientists most directly capable of doing harm. Regarding the promise and the perils of national biodefence programmes, the next chapter examines the case of the United States.

9 Biodefence

Lessons from the United States[1]

In the weeks following the attacks of 11 September 2001 in the United States, five Americans died after being deliberately infected with *B. anthracis* bacteria distributed through the postal system. Although the two sets of events were almost certainly of separate origin, in combination they generated intense fears of a future biological attack causing mass casualties. The US government had been aware of the increasing potential for biotechnology to be misused long before the anthrax attacks, and the Clinton administration had begun bolstering US biodefence capabilities in the late 1990s. In the 'post-9/11' atmosphere, however, annual federal government spending on biodefence programmes has increased enormously – from US$434 million in FY2001 to US$5.2 billion in FY2007. For the years FY2002–FY2007, the average amount spent on biodefence each year was around US$5.3 billion.[2]

US biodefence was once exclusively the domain of military agencies and was aimed at protecting battlefield troops against state-run BW programmes. Today, it is engaged in and promoted by a variety of government agencies contemplating 'bioterrorism', and it is aimed principally at protecting the American civilian population with pharmaceutical and other defences. Project BioShield, for example, allocates around US$6 billion over ten years to create a market for private companies to develop and sell to the US government the necessary vaccines and drugs to treat Americans in the event of a BW attack. The assumption behind a technology-driven policy like Project BioShield, and biodefence in general, is that it would in fact be possible to protect populations against an adversary bent on using biological agents. In the United States, this assumption is coupled with a strong belief that scientific research into vaccines and antimicrobial drugs can defeat every known select agent and the genetic permutations of each, and perhaps achieve defences applicable to entire categories of diseases.[3]

A key challenge, however, is that BW vaccines would only be useful in the highly unlikely event that the identity of the biological agent was known with certainty in advance of its use. At a congressional committee hearing in June 2005, Deputy Assistant Defense Secretary Dale Klein acknowledged that '[i]t's very difficult for us to come up with specific antidotes, pills and vaccines for everything the terrorists might throw at us'.[4] Notwithstanding this inherent shortcoming of pharmaceutical protection, pathogen research still has an important part to play in mitigating disease-based security risks. A 2004 report by the British Medical Association argued that

> though it is clearly impossible to cover all possible biological weaponry attacks that might occur as the revolution in modern biology progresses, there is every reason to make sensible preparation for dealing with relatively containable attacks using known agents.[5]

To the extent that pharmaceutical protection is worth pursuing, pathogen research conducted in the name of biodefence needs to be commissioned and conducted in a way that poses as few risks as possible to public health and safety, and to national and international security.

Most biodefence work is purely defensive and clearly benign: for example, development of biological detection systems; filtration, exclusion and decontamination procedures and systems for first responder training; medical facility outfitting; interagency communication and coordination; and epidemiological surveillance implementation. Such efforts bring the direct, practical benefits of reducing and possibly avoiding the human damage that would result from the use of BW. For the purposes of assessing disease-based security challenges, of greatest interest are those US biodefence projects which, although they might reduce the vulnerability of Americans, also pose risks to public health and safety, and to national and international security. Of particular concern are projects, conducted for 'threat-assessment' purposes, that investigate offensive BW capabilities. The US approach to biodefence is singled out for analysis not because it is the most problematic, but rather because it is the most conspicuous. It is possible that many of the challenges highlighted in this chapter are also relevant in countries that are less open and to which fewer scholars have turned their critical attention. This chapter explores three areas of particular concern. First, the opportunity costs associated with US pathogen research priorities measured in public health, scientific and biosecurity terms. Second, the legal problem of determining whether a BW programme is offensive or defensive in intent. And, third, the lessons and implications for East Asia of the US biodefence experience.

Research priorities and opportunity costs

In August 2003, *Nature* reported that US government scientists had developed a single-shot vaccine that protects monkeys from Ebola and that could eventually be used to protect humans.[6] In another experiment, USAMRIID scientists gave an experimental drug to monkeys that had been deliberately infected with Ebola. The disease is usually 100 per cent fatal in monkeys, but the drug caused one-third of the monkeys to survive.[7] US government sponsorship of Ebola research is part of a broader policy of promoting research on pathogens which, while dangerous, are not of ongoing importance for American public health. For example, on 9 May 2005 the National Institute for Allergy and Infectious Diseases (NIAID) announced its first grants under Project BioShield – approximately US$27 million was allocated to ten institutions to develop new therapeutics and vaccines against anthrax, botulinum toxin, Ebola, pneumonic plague, smallpox and tularaemia.[8] Although such grants bring the potential for greater scientific understanding of these diseases, prioritizing research in the field of potential BW agents also generates opportunity costs and security risks for the United States.

Competing public health concerns

On 30 September 2003, Boston University and the University of Texas at Galveston were each awarded US government grants of US$120 million to build a BSL-4 laboratory. In announcing the awards, Health and Human Services Secretary Tommy Thompson described them as 'a major step towards being able to provide Americans with effective therapies, vaccines and diagnostics for diseases caused by agents of bioterror as well as for naturally occurring emerging infections such as SARS and West Nile virus'.[9] Once built, the new laboratories will be capable of supporting research into emerging infectious disease agents, but there is little doubt that they will focus overwhelmingly on BW threats. It is a matter for debate within the United States whether the new money allocated to address potential BW threat agents is ultimately to the betterment of US public health. On the one hand, it is highly doubtful that the extra billions of dollars would have gone into infectious disease research anyway. According to NIAID director Anthony Fauci, biodefence research spending to jumpstart the invention of new vaccines, antibiotics and technologies for early diagnosis of disease has come on top of existing health budgets.[10] On the other hand, the prioritization of research on select agents over basic research on model micro-organisms like *E. coli* bacteria may well be hindering more valuable scientific breakthroughs. It is more difficult to work with select agents, not just because researchers are far less familiar with them, but also because they need to be handled in high-containment laboratories subject to strict safety and security measures.

In early 2005, 750 of the 1,143 scientists then in receipt of funding from the US National Institutes of Health wrote an open letter to the agency's head, Elias Zerhouni. They alleged that the NIH emphasis on biodefence research since 2002 had diverted researchers away from potential breakthroughs in basic research, and that research on select agents was crowding out research on micro-organisms that already pose a significant disease threat. The scientists claimed to be on the verge of making major breakthroughs in basic research on bacteria, which could then be transferred to more obscure pathogens such as select agents. They described as a misdirection of NIH priorities the 'diversion of research funds from projects of high public-health importance to projects of high biodefense but low public-health importance' and called on the NIH to create a new funding category for basic microbial science.[11] In reply to this letter, an editorial in the *Washington Post* disagreed with the scientists' judgement on public health:

> Security officials have stated repeatedly their belief that al Qaeda and others continue to search for more lethal bioweapons. Surely that makes biodefense projects of 'high public-health importance.' That this is not more widely understood means that there is still too little contact between the scientific community and national security and intelligence agencies.[12]

The latter view presently has the ascendancy in the United States because of heightened domestic concerns about 'terrorism' and a prevailing official assumption that non-state use of BW is a mass-casualty threat.[13] The danger, however, is that concentrating on select agent research may, in the longer term, diminish US capacity to resist infectious disease threats of deliberate or natural origin.

International collaboration

Beyond imposing scientific opportunity costs at home, the US preoccupation with security may also be hindering potentially valuable international collaborations on addressing infectious disease threats. Scientists in the United States have a proud history of collaborating with foreign colleagues to address infectious disease threats around the world. For example, USAMRIID has in the past sponsored research in Argentina to develop a vaccine against Argentine haemorrhagic fever (caused by the Junin virus), research in China on treating Korean haemorrhagic fever (caused by Hantaan virus) with the drug ribavirin, and research in Liberia on combating the Lassa fever virus also with ribavirin.[14] However, the new emphasis on researching agents that pose BW threats, combined with the recent tightening of US biosecurity regulations, has altered the way American scientists engage with the international scientific community. This could adversely affect the ability of the United States to address its own infectious disease problems and to provide much-needed US expertise to other parts of the world. An additional concern, according to Jeanne Guillemin, is that government-funded biodefence scientists are subject to the national security agenda regarding research decisions, and that this agenda gives priority to US interests over all other considerations.[15] If indeed this is the case, there is potential for conflict between narrowly defined goals of national security and the international character of American science and medicine.

From a US perspective, a principal security concern regarding international collaborations is that training people from foreign countries might increase the risk of pathogen misuse. For example, many of the scientists that filled important positions in Iraq's former BW programme received their advanced degrees in Britain and Germany before returning home.[16] The USA PATRIOT Act stipulates that any researcher from countries said to be aiding or abetting 'terrorists' is not allowed to handle select agents in the United States, regardless of whether he or she has a clean record. And President Bush's October 2002 Presidential Decision Directive (PDD-2) allows the US government to 'prohibit certain international students from receiving education and training in sensitive areas, including areas of study with direct application to the development and use of Weapons of Mass Destruction'.[17]

A possible opportunity cost of accentuating the national security dimension of pathogen research in the United States is that this will undermine the international collaborations upon which US science and security depend so heavily. The US biodefence programme itself builds upon advances made in a global network of scientists. US biologists collaborate with colleagues worldwide, attending meeting and presenting research at international meetings. And within the United States there is considerable reliance on foreign scientific talent and expertise. Tempering international collaborations with security measures necessarily creates a dilemma. On the one hand, it would be embarrassing for a US agency to be funding work in a foreign facility that was connected to the deliberate dispersal of a pathogen. On the other hand, tightened security requirements could stifle cooperation and make American collaborations unwelcome in many developing countries. Already, there is cause for researchers based outside the United States to hesitate before assuming the added cost and risk of working with US-based scientists as opposed to scientists located in a country with less stringent standards.

More research, greater risks

Research priorities for US biodefence, in addition to generating possible opportunity costs in terms of public health and international collaboration, also increase the risk of outbreak events inside the United States itself. More laboratories for investigating pathogens and potential therapies might reduce the vulnerability of Americans to infectious disease threats of deliberate or natural origin, but they also pose risks to health, safety and security. A major concern is that the expansion of laboratory research is taking place too quickly, with insufficient trained staff to operate all the new laboratories, and without adequate safeguards. Under such circumstances, accidents and security breaches are more likely.

Since the anthrax envelope attacks of 2001, the US biodefence programme has increased significantly in both scale and scope to involve multiple government agencies and a large number of contractors at universities and in industry. This is reflected, for example, in the make-up of NIH research grants. The number of grants for projects involving anthrax rose from 28 in 2000 to 253 in 2003. And, in 2000, 25 projects mentioned 'bioterrorism' and related words, compared to 665 in 2003.[18] At present there are four fully operational BSL-4 laboratories in the United States engaged in biodefence research: at the CDC in Atlanta, Georgia; at USAMRIID in Frederick, Maryland; at the Southwest Foundation for Biomedical Research in San Antonio, Texas; and at the NIH at Bethesda, Maryland. NIAID has allocated funds to construct two National Biocontainment Laboratories (NBLs) and nine Regional Biocontainment Laboratories (RBLs). The NBLs will reportedly contain BSL-4 laboratories but the RBLs will only go up to BSL-3. In addition, NIAID plans to build two BSL-4 laboratories for its own purposes, and the US Army and Department of Homeland Security also plan to construct additional laboratories.[19] Supporters of this expansion argue the October 2001 anthrax attacks exposed a shortage of the specialized, high-containment laboratory space needed to conduct research on micro-organisms that could be used as weapons, as well as on potential vaccines and therapies. The additional laboratories could also be useful for the purpose of safely researching agents that cause natural outbreaks of emerging and re-emerging infectious diseases, although US government justifications for expanded capabilities have emphasized BW threats.

However, the multi-billion-dollar project to keep America safe from outbreak events arguably increases the risk. It matters little that the US government says the pathogen research it sponsors is intended for defensive purposes – high-level stated intentions do not eliminate the dangers inherent in having large numbers of scientists engaged in such work. As of June 2004, more than 11,000 individuals and over 300 laboratories in the United States had reportedly received government approval to conduct experiments involving select agents.[20] With so many people and places involved in biodefence, there is an increased chance that pathogens might leak accidentally from a laboratory or be deliberately misused by a scientist. Safety and security in biodefence programmes are therefore of paramount importance lest efforts to circumvent an outbreak event become the source of one. Regarding biosafety risks, it is cause for concern that many inexperienced researchers have suddenly commenced work at facilities around the United States on projects involving select agents. A study by the Sunshine Project found that 97 per cent of principal investigators who received NIAID grants from 2001 to 2005 to study six pathogens (anthrax, brucellosis, glanders, plague, melioidosis or tularaemia) were newcomers to such research. Critics argue that giving work to these so-called 'bug jockeys' increases the risks of accidental pathogen release.[21]

In addition to safety considerations, more research on pathogens also increases the risk that potential BW agents might be diverted and misused. In 2004, the NAS called for greater biosecurity measures because it regarded biodefence research as 'precisely the sort of research likely to pose the most severe dual use dilemmas'.[22] Some biosecurity problems are associated with entire institutions – for example, the Los Alamos National Laboratory in New Mexico. In May 2003, US Department of Energy Inspector General Gregory Friedman testified that Los Alamos 'could not provide adequate assurance that classified, sensitive, or proprietary information was appropriately protected'.[23] More generally, biodefence research carries biosecurity risks associated with individual scientists. An increasing number of Americans are being granted access to dangerous pathogens and training in how to handle them. The danger is that the United States could be inadvertently creating its own training ground for would-be perpetrators of biological attacks. More than 11,000 people who work in government-certified microbiology laboratories have been cleared by the FBI, which checked them against criminal and terrorist databases.[24] However, pre-employment checks do not eliminate the possibility of a laboratory scientist deciding to misuse biological agents during the course of his or her employment.

Beyond generating biosafety and biosecurity risks, particular US biodefence priorities also pose risks measured in terms of international security. The next section concentrates on pathogen research carried out for 'threat-assessment' purposes, its status under international law and its implications for BW proliferation.

International law and the problem of intent

In 1973, the Soviet Politburo established Biopreparat. To the outside world, this was a state-owned pharmaceutical complex developing vaccines for the civilian market. In fact, Biopreparat was a military-funded programme for developing new types of BW.[25] An offensive BW programme could be easily concealed beneath a defensive disguise because of the dual-use nature of pathogenic micro-organisms. One example is the development and production of a vaccine, the most common form of which is an inactivated component of the target micro-organism itself. Producing doses for thousands of individuals necessarily involves growing a pathogen in large quantities. But the technologies and equipment required to do so could readily be turned to the mass production of BW agents for offensive purposes. In the United States at present, a grey area between offence and defence is the exploration of the potential of pathogens to be used as weapons in order to develop appropriate countermeasures. Such a policy, although probably peaceful in its intent, nevertheless risks breaching international law and stimulating 'defensive' BW proliferation in other countries. To assess this proposition, it is useful to explore four issues:

1   the potential for threat-assessment projects to contravene the BWC;
2   possible past US breaches of the Convention;
3   the genetic engineering of novel pathogens; and
4   biodefence programme transparency and proliferation risks.

Threat assessment

At the Los Alamos National Laboratory in New Mexico, scientists have built elaborate computer models of cities and then simulated the fallout from a hypothetical 'terrorist' attack. Simulations of smallpox releases in a major city have focused debate between proponents of targeted vaccinations and mass vaccination. In July 2005, a scientist on the smallpox simulation project, James Smith, told the *Washington Post* '[w]e're trying to be the best terrorists we can be. Sometimes we finish and we're like, "We're glad we're not terrorists."' If ever these simulations got into the wrong hands, Smith said, '[i]t would be a terrorist recipe for doing something terrible.'[26] Computer modelling of a smallpox event does not contravene international law, although the Los Alamos example illustrates how information obtained in the interests of defence could be used for offensive purposes.

Research and development projects on BW 'threat assessment' involve experimenting with offensive applications of pathogens so as to determine appropriate countermeasures – a practice known as 'red teaming'. However, such projects carry a security risk. On the one hand, against a specific biological threat, experimentation for threat-assessment purposes might on balance be worth that risk. And ethical justifications for such research might be strong. That is, faced with a specific threat, could the consciences of scientists and policy-makers tolerate not doing as much as they could to prepare? On the other hand, threat assessments might push beyond the bounds of international law and so damage operative moral norms as to make BW threats more numerous, not less. In order to develop defences against a putative BW agent, it is necessary to understand: the underlying mechanisms for pathogenicity, including infectivity and virulence; the way in which a microorganism evades the human immune system or acquires resistance to antibiotics; and the ways in which the agent may be dispersed, and its infectivity by each route. However, an understanding of these factors is also exactly what would be required for the development of BW.

Article I of the BWC prohibits development, production and stockpiling of BW but is silent on the question of research. In accordance with National Security Decision Memorandum 35, issued by National Security Advisor Henry Kissinger on 25 November 1969, the United States interprets its responsibilities under the BWC as permitting 'research into those offensive aspects of bacteriological/biological agents necessary to determine what defensive measures are required'.[27] The memorandum did not specify what types of research were justified for defensive purposes. On 23 December 1975, National Security Advisor Brent Scowcroft issued a second memorandum authorizing 'vulnerability studies' as permissible under the BWC, but no express authority for the creation of novel pathogens or weaponization techniques for threat-assessment purposes was cited.[28] In May 1989, however, in testimony before the US Senate Committee on Government Affairs, USAMRIID commander David Huxsoll stated that research to produce more virulent agents, to stabilize agents and on dissemination methods was prohibited by the BWC.[29]

Such comments by a US military officer today would not reflect the apparent attitude of his or her government regarding what constitutes defensive work. At present, a number of US government agencies are undertaking or plan to carry out research in exactly the areas cited by Huxsoll. Most prominent among these is the National Biodefense Analysis and Countermeasures Center (NBACC). Due to be completed in 2008, it is intended to provide the United States with high-containment laboratory space for biological threat characterization and bioforensic research. According to the US Department of Homeland Security, NBACC will form part of the National Interagency Biodefense Campus at Fort Detrick, Maryland, alongside NIAID and USAMRIID facilities. Its programmes will investigate the infectious properties of biological agents, the effectiveness of countermeasures and decontamination procedures, and techniques of forensic analysis. Part of NBACC is the Biological Threat Characterization Center, which will conduct laboratory experiments aimed at filling in information gaps on current and future biological threats. The Center will also assess vulnerabilities, conduct risk assessments and determine potential impacts in order to guide the development of countermeasures such as detectors, vaccines, drugs and decontamination technologies.[30] The CIA has reportedly assigned to NBACC at least one member of the 'Z-Division', a group jointly operated with Lawrence Livermore National Laboratory that specializes in analysing and duplicating weapons systems of potential adversaries.[31]

Many of the activities to be undertaken by NBACC could readily be interpreted by outsiders as the development of BW under the guise of threat assessment. In particular, weaponization feasibility studies and the engineering of novel pathogens arguably contravene the BWC. In a February 2004 presentation, George Korch, Deputy Director of NBACC, revealed that one of its research units intended to pursue a range of topics including 'aerosol dynamics', 'novel packaging', 'novel delivery of threat', 'genetic engineering' and 'red teaming'. At one point in his presentation, Korch summarized the threat-assessment task areas as: 'Acquire, Grow, Modify, Store, Stabilize, Package, Disperse.'[32] Such language is identical to that which would describe the functions of an offensive BW programme. Indeed, a 1998 report from the Office of the US Under Secretary of Defense for Acquisition and Technology stated: 'Stabilization and dispersion are proliferation concerns because these technologies increase the efficacy of biological agents.'[33] And, in light of the planned NBACC activities as described by Korch, a 2005 US State Department report which assessed that 'China maintains some elements of an offensive BW capability in violation of its BWC obligations' appeared to reflect an American double standard on BW when it warned that:

> From 1993 to the present, [Chinese] military scientists have published in open literature the results of studies of aerosol stability of bacteria, models of infectious virus aerosols, and detection of aerosolized viruses using polymerase chain reaction technology. Such advanced biotechnology techniques could be applicable to the development of offensive BW agents and weapons.[34]

By comparison, the 2006 Report to Congress by the US Chemical and Biological Defense Program (CBDP) reveals that facilities at the US Army Edgewood Chemical Biological Center include: 'Aerosol simulation chambers and the Aerodynamic Research Laboratory, comprising approximately 11,000 ft^2 of experimental aerodynamic facilities that include four wind tunnels for component and materials tests.'[35] In addition, the US Army Dugway Proving Ground has a Life Sciences Test Facility with multiple live biological agent test chambers at the BSL-3 level with aerosolization capability, and an Ambient Breeze Tunnel for biological stimulant system tests.[36] Such facilities could likewise be 'applicable to the development of offensive BW agents and weapons'.

To demonstrate exactly how a BW threat-assessment project might contravene international law, the next section weighs the details of three past US projects against the prohibitions contained in Article I of the BWC.

Putative US breaches of the BWC

In September 2001, the *New York Times* revealed the existence of three classified US biodefence projects. From 1997 to 2000, Project Clear Vision involved building and testing a Soviet-model bomblet for dispersing bacteria. In 1999–2000, Project Bacchus investigated whether a would-be 'terrorist' using commercially available materials and equipment could assemble an anthrax production facility undetected by the US and foreign governments. And, in early 2001, Project Jefferson involved the reproduction of a vaccine-resistant strain of anthrax bacteria.[37] The article's authors – Judith Miller, Stephen Engelberg and William Broad – had presumably known about these projects for several months already because they soon afterwards published a book containing more details.[38] An important caveat to what follows is that the work of these authors appears to be the only publicly available source regarding these three named projects.

Assessing the legality of these projects requires close attention to the precise wording of Article I of the BWC:

> Each State Party to this Convention undertakes never in any circumstances to develop, produce, stockpile or otherwise acquire or retain:
>
> 1   Microbial or other biological agents, or toxins whatever their origin or method of production, of types and in quantities that have no justification for prophylactic, protective or other peaceful purposes;
> 2   Weapons, equipment or means of delivery designed to use such agents or toxins for hostile purposes or in armed conflict.

Clear Vision

Of the three projects, the one most likely to have contravened the BWC was Clear Vision. This involved tests of bacteria bomblets, built according to a

Soviet design, and conducted by Battelle, a military contractor in Columbus, Ohio. The bomblets were reportedly filled with simulant pathogens and tested for their dissemination characteristics and reliability under different atmospheric conditions. Experiments in a wind tunnel revealed how the bomblets, after being released from a warhead, would fall on targets.[39] Before the testing took place, some US government legal experts had argued the experiments were not a breach of the BWC provided they were not intended for offensive purposes. Other officials argued that a weapon was, by definition, meant to inflict harm and therefore crossed the boundary into offensive work: 'A bomb was a bomb was a bomb.'[40]

Indeed, on a close reading of Article I, there is a strong case to be made that the BWC bans delivery systems *categorically*, whether intended for defensive purposes or not. Article I, paragraph (1), of the Convention permits the use of biological agents or toxins of types and in quantities justified for 'prophylactic, protective and other peaceful purposes'. This phrase is generally construed to include the development of pharmaceutical and other defences against biological attacks. Paragraph (2), however, is worded differently. It prohibits 'weapons, equipment or means of delivery designed to use such agents or toxins for hostile purposes or in armed conflict'. The difference between the words 'designed' and 'intended' is critical, such that paragraph (2) necessarily refers to the engineering features of a physical object rather than the intent of its user. For example, a person might *intend* to use a rifle for the peaceful purpose of stirring a tin of paint, but the rifle itself is *designed* for the hostile purpose of firing bullets. There is no provision in Article I for delivery mechanisms to be justified for 'prophylactic, protective and other peaceful purposes', and paragraph (2) does not contemplate delivery mechanisms being *intended* for hostile purposes.

The drafting of international treaties is an arduous process involving careful and deliberate choices of language. It is therefore significant that paragraphs (1) and (2) of Article I are written differently. Former US ambassador James Leonard, who led the original US negotiations of the BWC, has explained why the language of Article I with regard to delivery devices is more restrictive. According to Leonard, the BWC was never intended to legitimize the development and production of delivery devices for defensive purposes. If it had been, countries would all along have been able to develop and build the components for an entire weapon in the name of defence.[41] Such an interpretation is supported by the Preamble to the BWC, which contains this statement: 'The States Parties to this Convention ... [are] Determined for the sake of all mankind, to *exclude completely the possibility* of bacteriological (biological) agents and toxins being used as weapons' (emphasis added). The restrictive interpretation of Article I was adopted in draft recommendations for a biodefence code of conduct distributed by a group of NGOs to delegations attending the resumed session of the Fifth BWC Review Conference in November 2002. The NGOs argued that it is not permissible, even for defensive purposes, to construct delivery mechanisms designed for hostile use, whether or not hostile use is intended at the time of construction.[42]

Although a weaponization project like Clear Vision would be outside the limits of the BWC, it could nevertheless be considered legal under US domestic law. Under Title 18, section 175 of the United States Code, the development, production, stockpiling, transfer, acquisition, retention or possession of any biological agent, toxin or delivery system for use as a weapon is prohibited. However, the legislation defines the term 'for use as a weapon' to exclude 'the development, production, transfer, acquisition, retention, or possession of any biological agent, toxin, or *delivery system* for prophylactic, protective, or other peaceful purposes' (emphasis added). In other words, the US legislation, irrespective of international treaty obligations, contemplates 'peaceful' delivery systems. The difference in wording compared to that of Article I of the BWC may well have led some US officials to believe there was nothing wrong with Project Clear Vision.

Bacchus

Project Bacchus (named after the Roman god of fermentation) reportedly built a functioning facility that turned out two pounds of *B. anthracis* simulants: *B. thuringiensis* and *B. globigii*. Dried particle diameters ranged from 1 to 5 microns – the size most suitable for inhalation – and, as the journalists who revealed the existence of this project observed, '[i]f anthrax spores had been dropped into the fermenters, the United States could have made enough biological agent to mount a deadly attack'.[43] On a favourable reading of Article I of the BWC, emphasizing the words in paragraph (1), Bacchus produced a harmless *type* of biological agent in small *quantities* and therefore plausibly had the *peaceful purpose* of investigating the capabilities of potential enemies of the United States. Another reading, emphasizing paragraph (2), might be that, regardless of whether the biological agents used were harmless, the United States had produced *equipment* that was *designed* to use biological agents for *hostile* purposes. In effect, the United States had assembled everything necessary to produce BW short of an actual micro-organism capable of causing disease in humans. This means the BWC legality of Bacchus is at best questionable.

Jefferson

Closer to being permissible under the BWC was Project Jefferson. This involved experiments to reproduce the results of Russian research, as published by *Vaccine* in 1997, that had created a vaccine-resistant strain of anthrax bacteria. The researchers had inserted genes from *B. cereus* into *B. anthracis* bacteria, making them highly lethal against hamsters inoculated with Russia's standard anthrax vaccine.[44] The US officials involved in Project Jefferson were reportedly mindful of the BWC and the need for defensive intent.

Accordingly, the project was to produce only small quantities (one gram or less) of the modified anthrax bacteria.[45] The relevant BWC wording is contained in Article I, paragraph (1). On one interpretation, Project Jefferson had *produced* a biological agent capable of evading a vaccine and was therefore of a *type* which, in *quantities* however small, had no peaceful purpose. However, a more favourable reading of the Convention, and that which is probably most fair, is that the project *re*-produced a *type* of biological agent for the *protective* purpose of developing countermeasures against a known threat. By the same reasoning, however, there may be doubts about whether a 'peaceful purpose' was behind any military-linked effort to produce a *new* agent that had not already appeared in the scientific literature. On this point of doubt turns the BWC legality of some US biodefence research into genetically modified pathogens.

Genetic engineering of pathogens

The creation of 'recombinant' micro-organisms results from the isolation, insertion, deletion and modification of genetic material within a species of micro-organism and the movement of material from one species to another. This technology has already brought many benefits to medicine and has great potential to bring more in the future. One example is a new vaccine-production method called 'reverse genetics' that might enable public health authorities to respond more rapidly to evolving influenza threats. Through genetic engineering, the influenza virus's genome is converted from RNA to DNA, manipulated to remove the genes thought to cause pathogenicity, and converted back to RNA for vaccine production. From a security perspective, the kind of genetic engineering of most concern is that which makes pathogenic micro-organisms more dangerous. On the one hand, the production of an 'enhanced' pathogen can be for a genuinely peaceful purpose. A scientist might, for example, set out deliberately to generate a bacterium resistant to a certain class of antibiotics to determine whether it *could* become resistant to that class. Such information would be relevant to recommendations on how best to administer the antibiotic and could help to guide clinical infectious disease management. On the other hand, genetic engineering might enable a pathogen to defeat the defences erected by the human immune system and supplemented by existing medical technologies.

To address so-called 'emerging threats', the US government is sponsoring research into modified biological agents that might be used deliberately. For example, the CBDP is presently engaged in '[s]tudies to elucidate the toxicity and mechanism of action of non-traditional agents, and to determine the effectiveness of current medical countermeasures'.[46] Under the category of 'Genetically Engineered Threats', the goal of CBDP research is 'to assemble and integrate databases of protein domains responsible for lethality, delivery into human cells, evasion of the immune system, and therapeutic resistance'.[47] According to the programme's 2005 report to Congress, '[t]he direct payoff from the Emerging Threats capability investment is the prevention and/or mitigation of illness or injury following exposure to new, emerging and genetically modified CBW agents'.[48] To a more sceptical observer, however, the United States is also acquiring knowledge that could drive an offensive BW programme using genetically engineered pathogens to evade medical and pharmaceutical defences.

The declared policy of the US Department of Defense has clearly changed since 1989 when USAMRIID commander David Huxsoll commented: 'It would be absurd for us to create disease-causing organisms just to test therapies we develop.'[49] It used to be the case that US researchers conducted tests in cooperation with the host governments of countries where naturally occurring infectious diseases, thought to be also of BW concern, were already claiming victims. Perceived security risks and a pre-existing threat to human health clearly overlapped. For example, when Thomas Butler went to Tanzania to test antibiotics against plague, he did so in the context of a natural outbreak – his work addressed a known, ongoing threat. Similarly, when Project Jefferson produced a vaccine-resistant, genetically modified biological agent, it was only reproducing something that had already turned up in the scientific literature. It is a different matter to produce modified pathogens that no one, potential adversary or otherwise, has ever created.

Arguably, when a microbial threat exists only in a scientist's imagination, an experiment to create such a microbe is both unnecessary and overly risky. In the United States, some novel pathogens exist as disease threats only because US scientists created them. In 2003, a team of scientists at St Louis University, led by Mark Buller, supported by a NIAID biodefence grant, repeated a previously published Australian experiment on mousepox[50] with the intention of developing a pharmaceutical countermeasure. In the experiment, mice infected with genetically modified mousepox virus recovered when treated with a combination of antiviral drugs. As mousepox is closely related to the *variola major* virus, the result led Buller's team to hope that a treatment against genetically engineered smallpox could be developed.[51] Later, however, the scientists went further by applying the mousepox enhancement technique to cowpox virus which, unlike mousepox, infects humans. The rationale was reportedly '[t]o better understand how easy or difficult it would be to apply the same kind of genetic engineering to the human smallpox virus and make it more lethal'.[52] Although such work has been justified as 'necessary to explore what bioterrorists might do', other scientists have questioned the utility and wisdom of enhancing viruses.[53]

A major problem with creating hypothetical pathogens for threat-assessment purposes is the difficulty of correctly predicting technological innovations by states or non-state actors. Faced with so many possibilities for genetically modifying micro-organisms, it probably makes little sense to design a specific defence against any single genetic variation. Without accurate intelligence, it would be impossible to know what kind of organism a determined adversary would try to make. In such a situation, research could be dictated *ad infinitum* by the imaginations of defence planners.[54] The United States would effectively be engaged in an arms race with itself. Another problem is that the mere existence of novel agents potentially increases disease-based security risks to the United States homeland, whether measured in biosafety or biosecurity terms. The accidental leak of a supervirus from a laboratory could trigger an outbreak event, and there is also the risk that novel pathogens and the know-how that created them could be stolen and misused for malicious purposes.

Finally, it is important to consider the significance of genetically modified pathogens in terms of international law. The 2005 CBDP report to the US Congress states that '[w]ork conducted in this area [Emerging Threats and Special Projects] will be guided by all applicable agreements, convention and treaties and is performed to provide defensive capability only'.[55] However, it is difficult to see how the creation of novel BW agents would not contravene Article I of the BWC under which member states undertake 'never in any circumstances to develop . . . biological agents . . . *of types and in quantities* that have no justification for prophylactic, protective, or other peaceful purposes' (emphasis added). As Susan Wright has argued:

> [i]f there is no evidence of a threat posed by, say, a genetically engi-
> neered strain of cowpox that attacks the immune system, then there is no
> reasonable justification for developing such an organism. Arguably, to do
> so crosses the line between defense and offense.[56]

Moreover, issues of legality aside, the creation of a new agent with BW potential might also have significance in terms of the balance of international power. Other countries, suspicious of US intentions, might feel compelled to reproduce made-in-America pathogens in order to develop countermeasures. For this reason Tucker advocates a norm-strengthening statement by the US president 'renouncing the prospective development of genetically modified micro-organisms with increased pathogenicity for threat-assessment purposes and urging all countries to follow suit'.[57]

Transparency and 'defensive' BW proliferation

In the area of scientific endeavour to address disease-based security threats, a key challenge for the United States is to pursue defences in a way that does not endanger the norm against deliberate disease, as embodied in the BWC. The importance of transparency was recognized in 1986 at the Second BWC Review Conference when member states agreed to specific CBMs. These were extended and elaborated in 1991 at the Third BWC Review Confer- ence in 1991. The CBMs include: exchange of data on research centres and high-containment laboratories; exchange of data on and descriptions of national biological defence programmes and associated facilities; declarations on vaccine-production facilities; exchange of information on unusual infectious disease outbreaks; encouragement of publication of experiment results and promotion of use of knowledge; active promotion of scientific contacts through international conferences, symposia, seminars and other forums for exchange; and declaration of legislation, regulations and other BWC implementation measures.[58]

On the whole, the annual CBM returns of BWC member states have been few in number and of poor quality. For some countries, non-participation in the CBM process might be the result of technical difficulties, insufficient personnel and limited resources. Other countries, however, might simply be eschewing transparency. In the case of the United States, there was no mention of Clear Vision, Bacchus or Jefferson in its CBM declarations before those projects were revealed by journalists in 2001. If similar projects had been carried out inside a designated 'rogue state', they would undoubtedly have been viewed by the United States and other Western countries as violations of the BWC. For this reason, the latter cannot afford to be complacent about non-Western perceptions of ostensibly defensive BW activities. As the British Medical Association recently acknowledged, 'some countries may not view the West as benign in general and some biotechnology work being carried out in the West as necessarily above suspicion'.[59] It is also worth noting the possibility that the former Soviet Union maintained its BW programme after signing the BWC in 1972 because it believed the United States intended to do likewise, notwithstanding President Nixon's 1969 renunciation decision. In his 1999 memoir, *Biohazard*, Soviet defector Ken Alibek reflected:

> We didn't believe a word of Nixon's announcement. Even though the massive US biological munitions stockpile was ordered to be destroyed, and some twenty-two hundred researchers and technicians lost their jobs, we thought the Americans were only wrapping a thicker cloak around their activities.[60]

The difficulty of determining BWC compliance lies in the extent to which it comes down to perceptions of a given state's intent. And because intent is difficult to gauge reliably, states naturally err on the side of caution by focusing on the capabilities of potential adversaries. Allaying BW suspicions therefore requires as much transparency as possible regarding such capabilities as is consistent with safeguarding national security, although the point at which consistency is reached would be a matter for debate. At the 2002 resumed session of the Fifth BWC Review Conference, a group of NGOs recommended that the results of biodefence activities might need to be kept confidential, but that secrecy concerning the types and locations of such activities should be disavowed.[61] A recent indication that the United States might be moving towards greater transparency is the publication online of its 2004 return on BWC CBMs.[62]

Beyond the legal issue of BWC compliance, transparency is also important for strategic reasons. Beginning with the Clinton administration, the United States has shifted its focus away from the problem of state-run BW programmes and towards concerns about biological attacks perpetrated by non-state actors. However, the dynamics of proliferation by states are still important today. For at least three reasons, the very existence of the US biodefence programme might induce other countries to imitate it – BW proliferation in a defensive guise. First, in the eyes of a highly suspicious adversary, the development of pharmaceutical defences might constitute an attempt to acquire protection for a nation's own military forces against a biological agent that the nation intends to use in a BW 'first strike'. Prior to the 1991 Gulf War, for example, one of the reported reasons why the US military became concerned about the use of *B. anthracis* was the discovery that Iraqi soldiers captured in a covert pre-war operation had immunity against anthrax.[63] Second, any close association between defensive BW work and existing military programmes can create nervousness in an outside observer. For example, the conduct of classified BSL-3 biodefence research at Lawrence Livermore and Los Alamos National Laboratories might cause other countries to be concerned about possible US offensive intent because these facilities have historically been used for nuclear weapons development.[64] Third, the risk of BW proliferation is exacerbated by US threat-assessment projects. In particular, rival nations might be concerned that American exploration of novel BW threats could generate scientific breakthroughs that put them at a strategic disadvantage.[65] The result could be a BW arms race.

In conducting defensive work on pathogens, so as to reduce the vulnerability of Americans to a biological attack, the United States needs urgently to become more sensitive to how that work may be perceived by others. A particular danger is that current and planned threat-assessment projects could be seen as breaches of the prohibitions contained in Article I of the BWC – and that danger appears more vivid in light of the possibility that the United States has already violated the Convention through similar projects in the past. At stake is the credibility of the United States as an adherent to the rule of international law and as a sincere opponent of deliberately causing disease. Absent credible transparency, the development of offensive capabilities for defensive purposes risks undermining the international norm against BW. This in turn paradoxically risks accelerating BW proliferation; thus the United States must ensure its countermeasures are not counterproductive.

Conclusion: lessons for East Asia

Defending against deliberate disease is not a priority in East Asia like it is in the United States. Rather, the most serious disease-based security threats faced by countries in the region are of natural origin and this strongly influences priorities for pathogen research. Nevertheless, some countries in East Asia have programmes specifically devoted to addressing BW threats. For example, in October 2003 Singapore established a new laboratory, the

Defence Medical and Environmental Research Institute, to study the impact of biological hazards on a soldier's ability to fight and survive in battle. South Korea's military conducts defensive biological research, including the development of vaccines against anthrax and smallpox, to counter a perceived BW threat from North Korea. And in Japan, following Aum Shinrikyo's sarin attack in 1995 and its prior attempts to disperse BW, there is now an increased focus on BW defences. In general, however, pathogen research in East Asia has dual applications – a reflection of the overlap and synergies between infectious disease challenges of natural and deliberate origin.

The conclusion to this chapter on biodefence considers the extent to which the US experience provides lessons for governments in East Asia and its implications for addressing disease-based security challenges generally in the region. In summary, the lessons from the US biodefence programme are:

- prioritizing research on pathogens thought to have BW potential draws resources and expertise away from other areas of public health concern;
- requirements that such research be conducted according to strict biosecurity rules might inhibit international scientific collaborations;
- an increase in the number of personnel and facilities working on dangerous pathogens generates greater risks in terms of biosafety and biosecurity;
- Pathogen research that explores offensive BW applications for threat-assessment purposes potentially contravenes the BWC;
- the use of genetic-engineering technology to create novel BW agents simply to see whether it can be done is of questionable scientific worth and probably breaches both the spirit and the letter of the BWC;
- transparency is important in a biodefence programme to minimize suspicions of offensive intent and thus reduce the chances of stimulating an international BW arms race – the challenge is to achieve an appropriate level of information exchange while overcoming the natural tendency of governments to assume security is enhanced by secrecy.

In the context of East Asia, the lessons from the US biodefence experience are particularly relevant in relation to:

1 the biosafety and biosecurity risks of conducting more pathogen research;
2 international collaborations; and
3 transparency on the part of governments.

With regard to the first issue, East Asia is presently experiencing an expansion of interest and investment in biotechnology driven by health challenges, security concerns and economic interests. Countries with biosafety measures in place need to ensure these extend to new laboratories – three recent cases of laboratory-acquired SARS infections have put the region on notice. As compared to the United States, biosecurity is generally weak in East Asia. A consequence of an expanding biotechnology sector is more people working with dangerous pathogens, so the region urgently requires measures to prevent pathogen diversion and misuse.

On the issue of international collaborations, Article X of the BWC requires member states in a position to do so to 'cooperate in contributing individually or together with other States or international organizations to the further development and application of scientific discoveries in the field of bacteriology (biology) for prevention of disease, or for other peaceful purposes.' At the Fifth BWC Review Conference in 2001, Thailand warned BWC member states against neglecting the concerns of developing countries in securing adequate technical cooperation to promote peaceful uses of biotechnology, such as for public health and agricultural purposes.[66] Acting in the spirit of Article X, and for humanitarian and security reasons, US scientists and government agencies play a prominent role in addressing disease threats in East Asia. As such, any reduction of US international collaborations on biosecurity grounds could have deleterious consequences for East Asia.

Two examples of valuable collaboration are as follows. First, on 22 July 2003, the US Health and Human Services Secretary and the South Korean Minister for Health and Welfare signed a memorandum of understanding (MOU) to promote enhanced bilateral cooperation in the areas of vaccines and infectious disease research. The MOU called for expanded collaboration in such areas as laboratory research, TB, vaccine-preventable and other infectious diseases, epidemic investigation and surveillance, chronic diseases, and occupational health and public health law, as well as BW threats. Specific actions agreed to include exchanges of scientists and trainees, and other coordinated scientific research programmes.[67] Second, in May 2004, the Regional Emerging Diseases Intervention (REDI) Centre opened in Singapore. Jointly established by the US and Singapore governments, REDI is intended to strengthen infectious disease surveillance and outbreak response capabilities. The Centre aims, through research and training, to be a resource for countries in the Asia-Pacific region as they respond to new disease threats, whether of natural or deliberate origin. And, by undertaking research on diseases of particular relevance to the region, including SARS, influenza and dengue, REDI is expected to facilitate the development of new vaccines, drugs and diagnostic tests.[68]

Lastly, the US biodefence experience yields lessons on the need for transparency on the part of governments. In the light of planned US BW threat-assessment projects and possible past breaches of the BWC, the most important lesson some countries in East Asia might draw is that the United States itself is a direct source of BW threats. However, just as the United States needs urgently to become more transparent in order to allay international suspicions, the same applies to its two designated BW suspects in East Asia: North Korea and China. That the former is opaque and reclusive is a continuing problem, although China – whose BW potential is greater than that of North Korea – has sought to be more open. For example, in the

1980s China supported the development and implementation of CBMs in the form of information exchanges between BWC member states. Since 1987, it has reported annually to the UN on BWC-related information in accordance with the decisions of BWC Review Conferences. And China participated actively in the negotiations commenced in 1995 for a BWC verification protocol.[69] Nevertheless, in spite of this apparent record of good faith on BW issues, China remains a BW suspect in the eyes of most Western countries. This problem is not likely to be overcome until the Chinese Communist Party is able to govern with greater transparency. At the same time, however, China is sensitive to what it regards as hypocrisy in Western demands that developing countries be more open about their biotechnology activities. At the Fifth BWC Review Conference in 2001, the leader of the Chinese delegation criticized those countries that lecture others on BWC obligations while remaining silent about their own relevant activities and facilities: 'this is like a man with a flashlight in hand only to cast light on others while he himself stays in the dark.'[70]

In the areas of biosafety, biosecurity, international collaboration and transparency, the US experience of biodefence has important lessons and implications for East Asia. Within the region, commercial, scientific and security factors are leading to an increase in the number of people and facilities engaged in research on pathogenic micro-organisms. If properly managed, this could be of great benefit in addressing disease-based security challenges. If not, those challenges are likely to intensify. Such is the promise and the peril of pathogen research.

10 Conclusion

A government-funded scientist tests devices for dispersing bacteria, while his colleague experiments with techniques for making a particular bacterium more dangerous. A virology student works in a laboratory where live virus samples are not stored safely. A businessman boards an international flight after having been infected with a virus unknown to medical science. A scientist in a military laboratory steals vials of deadly bacteria and sends them to her victims in envelopes. A member of a millenarian cult attempts aerosol dispersal of what he believes is a virulent strain of bacteria obtained from the natural environment. A hospital nurse wearing no protective gear is infected with a new subtype of influenza while caring for a sick poultry farmer. A senior army officer orders that plague-infected fleas be placed inside porcelain bombs to be dropped from aircraft onto towns and villages.

In each of these situations, the common thread is the potential for an outbreak event that causes a high degree of damage and disruption in a short space of time. Binding them together also are the synergies between infectious disease threats that occur through natural processes and those that arise as a result of human agency.

The senior army officer wages biological warfare in a part of the world where there are regular natural outbreaks of the disease he is trying to cause deliberately, so there may be doubts about whether an attack has occurred at all. The scientist testing bacteria dispersal devices could be helping his country to defend against a biological attack, such as the one planned by the member of the millenarian cult. Or he might use his position and knowledge to steal some bacteria for engaging in deliberate disease on his own. The scientist's colleague investigating the deadly properties of a pathogen could be seeking to develop a drug to treat the illness that pathogen would cause if spread deliberately. And similar research could be undertaken to investigate whether the influenza strain sickening the poultry farmer has the potential to spread between humans. The virology student working in the unsafe laboratory could be part of a team trying desperately to discover more about a mysterious new virus so as to improve the treatment of people it infects. But if the student is infected with the virus and transmits it to others, there could be an outbreak similar to the one started by the infected businessman boarding an international flight. The outbreak might be mistaken for a deliberate attack – but deliberate, accidental or naturally occurring, the public health imperatives of containing disease and treating patients are the same.

Every kind of actual and potential illness in humans is a health issue, although some threats to human health warrant special treatment because of their broader significance to security. The framework proposed by this book for elevating these to the security realm rests on three conceptual pillars:

1   dread of infection as an impetus towards treating infectious disease threats in security terms;
2   securitization limited to extreme threats in three overlapping dimensions (naturally occurring disease outbreaks, BW and the risks of research on pathogenic micro-organisms); and
3   designation of the state as the rallying point for responding to these threats.

East Asia is a worthy geographical arena for exploring this framework because the region has been, and is likely to remain, the cradle of emerging infectious diseases that spread rapidly, it has a history of state and non-state interest in and use of BW, and the number of people and facilities in East Asia engaged in pathogen research is increasing.

This concluding chapter, presented in three sections, draws together the major themes of the book. The first summarizes the security significance of naturally occurring and deliberately caused infectious disease outbreaks in East Asia. The second highlights public health as the most worthwhile response applicable to both of these threats. And the third section discusses the ongoing need to strive for balance between the promise and the perils, measured in public health and security terms, of research on pathogenic micro-organisms.

Natural plagues and biological weapons

At present, the most serious disease-based security challenge facing East Asia is an outbreak event of natural origin. In the aftermath of SARS, and at a time when an influenza pandemic is looming, it is becoming clear that some infectious disease threats, because of their capacity to cause a high degree of damage and disruption in a short space of time, ought not to be treated only as health issues. The security significance of the 2003 SARS outbreak lay in the unfamiliar and fast-moving nature of this disease. In East Asia, hospitals were overwhelmed, trade and tourism suffered, and people's visceral dread of contagion generated high levels of social disruption and occasional breakdowns in civil order. The response of governments in the region was to treat SARS as a first-order issue of national concern; one which attracted extraordinary interventions against an unforeseen and largely mysterious threat. The positive legacy of this outbreak event includes new disease surveillance and reporting techniques, expanded mechanisms for collaborative research on pathogenic micro-organisms, new procedures for infection control, and channels for informing and educating the public about health risks. In addition, the levels of emergency response required to defeat SARS and the media attention it generated have sensitized politicians and people in general to the threat posed by emerging infectious diseases. Moreover, the SARS experience may turn out to have been a valuable 'dress rehearsal' for responding to an outbreak event of far greater consequence – a pandemic of influenza. As was the case during the 2003 SARS outbreak, the burden of illness and death during an influenza pandemic would be compounded by the human dread of infection and the speed with which this disease would spread through countries and around the globe.

The security significance of the H5N1 avian influenza virus, which has predominantly affected birds in East Asia, lies in the danger that it could soon acquire human hosts on a global scale. In contrast to the experience of past pandemics, which were all the more damaging because they erupted with no warning, national governments and international health authorities around the world have an unprecedented window of opportunity to delay, curtail and mitigate a worldwide outbreak event. The main tasks are to reduce the risk of human infection with this new influenza virus subtype and to enhance health system capabilities for timely case detection and response if H5N1 (or another virus subtype with pandemic potential) starts transmitting between humans. And, against a microbial threat that knows no borders, countries that are presently not directly affected by avian influenza have a security interest in treating this problem as if it were their own. Risk reduction has so far included culling of infected birds and vaccination of those most likely to be infected. As of the end of 2006, however, this strategy appeared unlikely to succeed, especially if the poorer countries of East Asia did not receive increased international assistance. In any event, because early outbreaks of H5N1 in poultry were not contained, the virus has become endemic to the region and thus may be impossible to eradicate. In the face of an overdue (and possibly imminent) influenza pandemic, the most important means of preparing for damage control are laboratory-based disease surveillance and research, the acquisition and use of antiviral drugs and influenza vaccines, and communication between governments and the public regarding the risks posed by avian influenza. In the longer term, the best responses to future influenza pandemics are to expand world vaccine manufacturing capacity far beyond what presently exists and to ramp up the rate of vaccination against regular, seasonal influenza.

In addition to the threat of naturally occurring outbreak events, the problem of BW is a continuing disease-based security challenge in East Asia. To put this challenge in perspective, however, BW do not constitute as grave a threat to the health of individuals and the stability of states as pandemic influenza. And an assessment of the science and history of biological warfare and of the prospect of biological attacks by non-state perpetrators reveals that

BW are generally not a 'mass destruction' issue. For reasons related to biological agent choice and circumstances of delivery, BW effects are diverse in nature and scale. Using deliberate disease to achieve mass casualties would be considerably more difficult than using nuclear weapons. This book has therefore rejected the awkward paradigm of WMD – one that encourages the drawing of false comparisons between weapons categories based on fundamentally different scientific principles – and has instead proposed that solutions to the problem of BW are more likely to be found by recognizing the extensive overlap, for response purposes, between infectious disease outbreak events caused deliberately and those of natural origin.

Notwithstanding the tactical and strategic shortcomings of BW, this form of weaponry has nevertheless attracted the interest of state and non-state actors in the past and is likely to remain a security concern in East Asia. The region has a history of BW use (actual and alleged) and contains countries presently accused of BW possession. East Asia became the cradle of modern biological warfare when the Japanese general Shiro Ishii deployed weapons based on *Y. pestis* and other pathogenic micro-organisms on the Chinese mainland. Subsequent Cold War allegations of BW use on the Korean peninsula and in Myanmar have not been proven, but this itself illustrates one of the most important overlaps between deliberately caused and naturally occurring outbreak events: that it can be difficult to distinguish between the two. It is also difficult to determine whether a given country today possesses BW. The dual-use nature of BW-relevant agents, equipment and facilities means that accurate information about illicit activities is extremely difficult to obtain. This is well demonstrated by the inability of the US government to prove that its pre-Iraq War claims about an Iraqi BW programme were correct.

North Korea and China are routinely cited as BW suspects in East Asia; however, the evidence used to support this is inherently problematic. In particular, although intelligence assessments may indicate that a given country has the capability to produce potential BW agents (this could be said of most countries), it is extremely difficult to establish whether this is matched by intent to use them for non-peaceful purposes. North Korean defectors have described in some detail their country's past BW activities, so it is reasonable to suspect Pyongyang might retain some relevant materials and equipment. However, it is doubtful whether North Korea would ever want or need to use BW. The country's health system is ill-equipped to cope if a biological attack went wrong, if a BW facility suffered a biosafety or biosecurity breach or if an adversary decided to retaliate in kind. With regard to China, there is little evidence regarding the existence and nature of an offensive BW programme in the past. And, although published US intelligence assessments emphasize China's present capability to produce and use BW, they contain no evidence to indicate that this is matched by hostile intent.

Regarding the threat of BW attacks perpetrated by entities other than states, the record is mixed in East Asia. The Aum Shinrikyo cult in Japan ran the largest-ever non-state BW programme in the early 1990s, although it ultimately failed to cause a single BW casualty. And, although there is some evidence that Muslim militants in Southeast Asia have taken an interest in biological agents, it is unlikely that they would have the desire or resources to engage seriously in deliberate disease. On the whole, the threat of biological attacks perpetrated by non-state actors, both in East Asia and in general, is presently not great and should not be exaggerated. The most likely perpetrators of an attack resulting in mass casualties would be those with a religious motivation, an apocalyptic worldview envisaging disease as divine punishment, a high degree of relevant scientific expertise and large financial resources. At present, no known non-state organization possesses this configuration of attributes.

The alternative to building a BW capability from scratch, as Aum Shinrikyo attempted to do, would be to attract state sponsorship. However, a state concerned about its security and international reputation would be highly unlikely to risk bestowing such a capability on the kind of group most likely to be interested in launching biological attacks. And, without the sophisticated delivery mechanisms available from a state-run BW programme, infecting a target population with biological agents would be difficult. Agent delivery using crop dusters would generally fail to produce particles of a size suitable for inhalation, and epidemiological and motivational factors would militate against 'suicide sneezers' being a serious threat. The notion of *inadvertent* state sponsorship, however, is one that warrants further exploration. The FBI has yet to close the case of 'Amerithrax', although publicly available evidence suggests strongly that the United States was attacked by a US defence establishment insider using American-made anthrax bacteria.

The threat of BW-use by state or non-state actors in East Asia, although it appears less serious than the clear and present danger posed by a naturally occurring influenza outbreak, is nevertheless one that warrants careful monitoring. To guard against any erosion of the line between the capability to engage in deliberate disease and intent to do so, a range of responses are available. These include military, intelligence, legal and public health responses. The latter are the most valuable because of their applicability to outbreak events of both deliberate and natural origin.

Prioritizing public health

Regardless of the origin of an outbreak event, the public health imperatives of preventing and treating illness are the same. For this reason, broadly applicable measures aimed at limiting vulnerability to infectious disease threats are the most worthwhile area in which to invest financial resources and political attention. Within East Asia, the need to prioritize public health responses spans the region. Poorer countries such as Cambodia, Laos and Myanmar are particularly vulnerable to outbreak events occurring in their territory because of a paucity of health resources. Wealthier countries like

Japan, Singapore and South Korea are also vulnerable despite the higher standards of healthcare enjoyed by their citizens. This is largely because the public health systems of these countries, less accustomed to infectious disease threats, are ill-prepared for dealing with the morbidity, mortality and social anxiety burden of an outbreak event. And, in the case of China, the largest and most populous country in East Asia, its vulnerability to such an event stems largely from the fact that health resources are allocated so unevenly as to open up gaps in outbreak response capacity.

The effectiveness of public health responses to disease-based security threats would depend upon the strength of two main pillars. The first, highly sensitive and well-connected systems (local and global) for disease surveillance and response, would be a vital means of containing an outbreak in its early stages and facilitating the timely treatment of victims. The second, national health systems with surge capacity in areas such as medical care and diagnostics, would be better able to accommodate sudden increases in patient demand. At the domestic level, specific lessons from the SARS experience for dealing with outbreak events include the importance of preventing disease among essential health workers, the value of cooperation and communication across government sectors, and the need to pre-empt the possibility of the human dread of infection precipitating a breakdown in civil order. Moreover, there is an indispensable international dimension to public health responses; an outbreak event inside one country is potentially a problem for others, especially if the disease in question is contagious. In such circumstances, the East Asia region as a whole would be better able to resist infectious disease threats if wealthier countries worked to enhance the outbreak response capacity of poorer countries' health systems as well as their own. In addition, well-resourced countries closely connected to but outside East Asia, such as the United States and Australia, have an interest in ensuring the public health and security fallout from an outbreak event does not spread within and beyond the region.

Other categories of responses (military, intelligence and legal) to the threat of outbreak events are not as directly valuable, although they may play an important role in complementing public health responses. For example, in the context of responding to outbreak events, military personnel and resources could play an important supportive role in ensuring the security of medical supplies and facilities. In the area of legal responses to disease-based security challenges, the BWC is emerging as a 'dual-use' response to infectious disease threats arising both from human agency and as a result of natural processes. The advantage of the new process for reforming the BWC is that discussions among its member states are now less about making the Convention emulate verifiable regimes governing other weapons. Rather, the BWC could more usefully become part of an expanded response to the threat of outbreak events in general. In addition to maintaining the traditional role of the Convention as a ban on deliberate disease, the BWC member states have begun to recognize the importance to international security of strong mechanisms for infectious disease surveillance and outbreak response. Such recognition lends vital political support to the public health efforts of the hitherto weak WHO, and it complements the revised IHR under which this body is granted increased legal powers to address outbreak threats.

Pathogen research: striking a balance

The effectiveness of public health responses to actual and potential outbreak events, whether of deliberate or natural origin, is vitally supported by research on the origins, properties, behaviour and epidemiology of pathogenic micro-organisms. Within East Asia, the number of people and facilities engaged in pathogen research is increasing. If properly managed, such research could be of great benefit in addressing disease-based security challenges. However, where pathogenic micro-organisms are not handled and stored in a safe and secure manner, there is a higher risk of accidental outbreaks and the diversion of pathogens for non-peaceful purposes. Moreover, if some aspects of pathogen research are not conducted with an appropriate degree of transparency, there is an international security risk that this may encourage BW proliferation. As advances in biotechnology continue into the future, and as the biotechnology sector in East Asia expands, the ongoing challenge will be to strike a balance between the promise and the perils, measured in public health and security terms, of research on pathogenic micro-organisms.

An imbalance demanding urgent attention in East Asia, the rectification of which would pose few public health or security dilemmas, concerns the risk of accidental outbreak events. Although some countries already have comprehensive biosafety regimes in place based on international guidelines, the regulation of laboratory practices and containment standards in East Asia as a whole is insufficient. Three recent incidents in the region of laboratory workers being exposed to the SARS virus have highlighted the necessity for pathogen research to be conducted safely. Notwithstanding the additional administrative and financial costs of regulating biosafety in new and existing laboratories, this would be a relatively straightforward and uncontroversial response to the risks of pathogen research. A more complicated balancing issue that is likely to require constant monitoring is biosecurity. In general, across East Asia, there is an insufficient level of domestic regulation aimed at preventing the diversion and misuse of pathogens. However, the dilemma arises as to how much security regulation should be imposed on research which, for the most part, is intended to benefit humankind. The US experience of biosecurity regulation suggests that too great a concern for security on the part of governments may be counterproductive if it excessively hinders scientific advances with the potential to reduce human vulnerability to infectious disease threats. In particular, if the administrative and financial burdens associated with laboratory work on particular micro-organisms appear too great, and if the risks of personal legal liability are perceived as too high, many scientists may simply opt out of potentially life-saving pathogen research.

Emerging as a complement to government biosecurity regulation is the notion of security-oriented ethical guidelines for biological scientists. No matter that the intentions of such scientists may be entirely noble, advances in biotechnology are increasing the need for them to be more conscious of the security risks posed by their laboratory practices, research methods and experiment results. Codes of conduct, incorporating both top-down and bottom-up approaches to governance, would be a useful means of addressing the risk that biological scientists might deliberately or inadvertently contribute to malign misuses of pathogens. The security consciousness of scientists might, in some cases, extend to the point of deciding that some research should not be carried out at all. However, it is likely to be an ongoing balancing challenge to obtain agreement among scientists and other communities of interest on exactly when the advantages of particular research outweigh its dangers. For example, genetic engineering of pathogenic micro-organisms has proven to be a valuable means of addressing infectious disease threats of natural origin. However, this technology can also lead to the creation of agents that are more useful for BW purposes because of their stability, ease of delivery, infectivity and/or resistance to pharmaceutical defences.

The final challenge for balancing the promise and the peril of pathogen research relates to biodefence. This is presently not as high-profile an issue in East Asia as it is in the United States – at present, the most serious disease-based security threats faced by countries in the region are of natural origin. Nevertheless, if BW threats in the region become more prominent because of technological advancements and/or an erosion of the norm against deliberate disease, there is potential for national biodefence activities to commence or increase. The lesson from the US experience has been that, although biodefence brings some promise of reducing vulnerability to biological attacks through pharmaceutical protection, it also creates security pitfalls. Governments in East Asia looking to engage in biodefence should be mindful, for example, that prioritizing research on biological agents with BW potential can draw resources and expertise away from other areas of public health concern, and that increasing the number of personnel and facilities working on dangerous pathogens generates more biosafety and biosecurity risks.

The most significant balancing challenge for a prospective biodefence programme concerns international law and norms against deliberate disease, and the US experience is again a cautionary tale. A salient issue is that laboratory or field-scale research carried out for threat-assessment purposes carries a risk of breaching the BWC and exacerbating BW proliferation. On the one hand it could be argued that, against a specific biological threat, experimentation to investigate offensive applications would on balance be worth the security risk – indeed, a decision *not* to investigate could decrease the chance of being able to respond adequately against this specific threat if it were to occur. On the other hand, each experiment of this kind gradually erodes the norm against deliberate disease, and this in turn increases the overall likelihood of biological attacks. Two potential areas of BW threat-assessment are of particular concern. The first – projects to create pathogens that have not previously existed as an infectious disease threat – could be interpreted as the development of BW and should therefore be the subject of strict regulation and extraordinary transparency. The second – experimentation on the dispersal of pathogenic agents – is a step too far and ought not to be a part of a biodefence programme at all; the key to combating the problem of BW is to keep the 'biological' well separated from the 'weapon'.

Reflections on once and future plagues

For thousands of years, pathogenic micro-organisms have shaped the fortunes of humankind. Under the onslaught of countless plagues and poxes, individuals have perished, armies have crumbled and civilizations have retreated. Throughout most of human history, the origins and nature of infectious disease outbreaks were largely a mystery, with their devastating effects frequently attributed to supernatural forces. Under such circumstances, political leaders would have had little reason to suppose any actions other than prayer or sacrifice could make their people safe. By the late nineteenth century, breakthroughs in medical and biological research had led to the discovery of many microscopic organisms that cause disease. Thereafter, humans began to wage a science-based campaign against their primordial foes. Within decades, vaccines and antibiotics had brought about a temporary suspension of microbial threats in many parts of the world, and entire generations came to believe vulnerability to infectious diseases had been consigned to the dustbin of history. However, with the advent of microbiological knowledge and techniques came the potential for disease outbreaks to be caused deliberately and systematically. And, before the close of the twentieth century, the struggle against naturally occurring infectious disease had turned to addressing the emergence of diseases never before seen.

Today, the public health tasks of preventing and treating infectious disease continue. However, some disease threats are so serious that they warrant priority political attention, a higher level of resource allocation and the implementation of extraordinary response measures. Focusing on data from East Asia, and drawing lessons from experiences beyond the region, this book has advocated a new framework for securitizing infectious diseases. Beyond the morbidity and mortality burden they impose, outbreak events of deliberate, natural or accidental origin are a security concern because of the dread they inspire and the swiftness with which they cause damage and disruption. By understanding and harnessing the synergies between the threats posed by BW, natural outbreaks and pathogen research, the response to each is enhanced.

Once considered tools of the gods, and always a public health concern, infectious diseases also have the potential to threaten security. Looking into the future, advances in biotechnology are likely to bring new dangers as well as new benefits. And increases in global human connectedness, although they may facilitate the worldwide spread of disease, carry the promise of improved cooperative action against pathogenic micro-organisms. The greatest of human struggles goes on.

Notes

1 Infectious diseases as a security challenge

1 R. Paris, 'Human security: paradigm shift or hot air?', *International Security* 26, 2, 2001, 87–102, p. 95.
2 Full text of UNSCR 1308 (2000) available at: www.un.org/Docs/scres/2000/sc2000.htm.
3 NIC, *The Global Infectious Disease Threat and its Implications for the United States* (National Intelligence Council Online, January 2000). Online, available at: www.dni.gov/nic/special_globalinfectious.html (accessed 31 August 2006).
4 R.J. Jackson, A.J. Ramsay, C.D. Christensen, S. Beaton, D.F. Hall and I.A. Ramshaw, 'Expression of mouse Interleukin-4 by a recombinant ectromelia virus suppresses cytolytic lymphocyte responses and overcomes genetic resistance to mousepox', *Journal of Virology* 75, 3, 2001, 1205–1210.
5 J. Youde, 'Enter the fourth horseman: health security and international relations theory', *Whitehead Journal of Diplomacy and International Relations* 6, 1, 2005, 193–208, p. 194.
6 Ibid., p. 200.
7 Ibid., pp. 204–205.
8 See, for example, S. Elbe, *Strategic Implications of HIV/AIDS, Adelphi Paper 357*, New York: Oxford University Press, 2003; G. Prins, 'AIDS and global security', *International Affairs* 80, 5, 2004, 931–952; P.W. Singer, 'AIDS and international security', *Survival* 44, 1, 2002, 145–158.
9 For the purposes of this book, 'East Asia' comprises 15 countries: Brunei, Cambodia, China (and Taiwan), Indonesia, Japan, Laos, Malaysia, Myanmar, North Korea, Philippines, Singapore, South Korea, Thailand, Timor-Leste and Vietnam.
10 S. Szreter, 'Health and security in historical perspective', in *Global Health Challenges for Human Security*, L. Chen, J. Leaning and V. Narasimhan (eds), Cambridge, MA: Global Equity Initiative, Asia Center, Harvard University, 2003, p. 31.
11 Livy, *The War With Hannibal*, A.D. Selincourt (trans.), London: Penguin, 1965, pp. 331–332.
12 C. Coker, *War and Disease* (21st Century Trust Online, 2004). Online, available at: www.21stcenturytrust.org/coker2.html (accessed 12 December 2005).
13 E. Croddy, *Chemical and Biological Warfare: a Comprehensive Survey for the Concerned Citizen*, New York: Copernicus, 2002, pp. 249–250.
14 H. Zinsser, *Rats, Lice, and History*, London: Routledge, 1937, p. 165.
15 S. Selin, 'The security implications of SARS', *CANCAPS Bulletin* 37, 2003, 9–13, p. 10.
16 R.J. Evans, 'Epidemics and revolutions: cholera in nineteenth-century Europe', in *Epidemics and Ideas: Essays on the Historical Perception of Pestilence*, T. Ranger and P. Slack (eds), New York: Cambridge University Press, 1992, p. 159.

17 A.T. Price-Smith, *The Health of Nations: Infectious Disease, Environmental Change, and Their Effects on National Security and Development*, Cambridge, MA: MIT Press, 2002, p. 128.

18 G.H. Brundtland, *New Global Challenges: Health and Security from HIV to SARS* (WHO Online, 18 July 2003). Online, available at: www.who.int/dg/brundt-land/speeches/2003/genevasecuritypolicy/en/print.html (accessed 6 January 2005).

19 Coker, *War and Disease* (URL cited).

20 This book is concerned only with BW directed at human targets. For an excellent discussion of anti-crop and anti-animal BW programmes, see chapters 10 and 11 respectively of M. Wheelis, L. Rozsa and M. Dando (eds), *Deadly Cultures: Biological Weapons since 1945*, Cambridge, MA: Harvard University Press, 2006.

21 MIIS, *Chemical and Biological Weapons: Possession and Programs Past and Present* (Monterey Institute of International Studies Online, 9 April 2002). Online, available at: cns.miis.edu/research/cbw/possess.htm (accessed 1 September 2006).

22 C. McInnes, 'Health and security studies', in *Health, Foreign Policy and Security* A. Ingram (ed.), London: Nuffield Trust, 2004, pp. 44–46.

23 Ibid., p. 49.

24 See P. Chalk, 'Disease and the complex process of securitization in the Asia-Pacific', in *Non-Traditional Security in Asia: Dilemmas in Securitisation*, M. Caballero-Anthony, R. Emmers and A. Acharya (eds), Aldershot: Ashgate, 2006; S. Elbe, 'Should HIV/AIDS be securitized? The ethical dilemmas of linking HIV/AIDS and security', *International Studies Quarterly* 50, 1, 2006, 119–144.

25 B. Buzan, O. Waever and J.d. Wilde, *Security: a New Framework for Analysis*, London: Lynne Rienner, 1998, pp. 23–24.

26 O. Waever, 'Securitization and desecuritization', in *On Security*, R.D. Lipschutz (ed.), New York: Columbia University Press, 1995, p. 57.

27 Buzan, Waever and Wilde, *Security*, p. 5.

28 B. Buzan, *People, States and Fear: an Agenda for International Security Studies in the Post-Cold War Era*, 2nd edn, London: Harvester Wheatsheaf, 1991, p. 115; Buzan, Waever and Wilde, *Security*, p. 25.

29 P. Slovic, B. Fischhoff and S. Lichtenstein, 'Facts and fears: understanding perceived risk', in *Societal Risk Assessment: How Safe is Safe Enough?* R.C. Schwing and W.A. Albers (eds), New York: Plenum, 1980, p. 209.

30 Ibid., p. 211.

31 WHO, *World Health Report 2002: Reducing Risks, Promoting Healthy Life*, World Health Organization, 2002, p. 32.

32 H. Schell, 'Outburst! A chilling true story about emerging-virus narratives and pandemic social change', *Configurations* 5, 1, 1997, p. 96.

33 Ibid., p. 112.

34 J. Stern, 'Dreaded risks and the control of biological weapons', *International Security* 27, 3, 2002, p. 102.

35 Price-Smith, *The Health of Nations*, pp. 15–16.

36 R. Chandavarkar, 'Plague panic and epidemic politics in India, 1896–1914', in *Epidemics and Ideas: Essays on the Historical Perception of Pestilence*, T. Ranger and P. Slack (eds), New York: Cambridge University Press, 1992, pp. 203–204.

37 Buzan, *People, States and Fear*, p. 117.

38 R. Ullman, 'Redefining security', *International Security* 8, 1, 1983, p. 133.

39 A.J. Bellamy and M. McDonald, ' "The utility of human security": which humans? What Security? A reply to Thomas and Tow', *Security Dialogue* 33, 3, 2002, p. 374.

40 UN, *A More Secure World: Our Shared Responsibility. Report of the High-Level Panel on Threats, Challenges and Change*, United Nations, 2004, p. 19.

41 Chandavarkar, 'Plague panic and epidemic politics in India', pp. 204, 208–210.
42 See Price-Smith, *The Health of Nations*, pp. 16–17.
43 C. McInnes 'Health and security studies', in *Health, Foreign Policy and Security*, A. Ingram (ed.). London: Nuffield Trust, 2004, p. 54.
44 Y.S. Wong and G. Chan, *The SAF SARS Diaries*, Singapore Armed Forces, 2004, p. 33.
45 Ibid.
46 McInnes, 'Health and security studies', p. 53.
47 UN, *A More Secure World*, p. 14.
48 D.P. Fidler, *Germs, Norms and Power: Global Health's Political Revolution* (Law, Social Justice & Global Development Online, 4 June 2004). Online, available at: www2.warwick.ac.uk/fac/soc/law/elj/lgd/2004_1/fidler/ (accessed 19 September 2006).
49 W. Orent, 'An "illegal" outbreak of plague', *Los Angeles Times* 8 August 2004, M1.
50 Elbe, 'Should HIV/AIDS be securitized?', p. 119.
51 See E. Emanuel and A. Wertheimer, 'Who should get influenza vaccine when not all can?', *Science* 312, 5775, 2006, 854–855.
52 C. McInnes and K. Lee, 'Health, security and foreign policy', *Review of International Studies* 32, 1, 2006, 5–23, p. 11.
53 D. Yach, S.R. Leeder, J. Bell and B. Kistnasamy, 'Global chronic diseases', *Science* 307, 5708, 2005, 317.
54 Ibid.
55 L. Wang, L. Kong, F. Wu, Y. Bai and R. Burton, 'Preventing chronic diseases in China', *The Lancet* 366, 9499, 2005, 1821–1824.
56 H. Feldbaum and K. Lee, 'Public health and security', in *Health, Foreign Policy and Security*, A. Ingram (ed.). London: Nuffield Trust, 2004, p. 22.
57 R. Thakur, 'From national to human security', in *Asia-Pacific Security: The Economics-Politics Nexus*, S. Harris and A. Mack (eds). Sydney: Allen & Unwin, 1997, pp. 53–54.
58 Human Security Centre, *Human Security Report 2005: War and Peace in the 21st Century*, University of British Columbia, 2005, p. viii.
59 UNDP, *Human Development Report*, United Nations Development Program, 1994.
60 A. Acharya, 'Human security: what kind for the Asia-Pacific?', in *The Human Face of Security: Asia-Pacific Perspectives*, D. Dickens (ed.), Canberra Paper on Strategy and Defence No. 144, Canberra: Australian National University, 2002, p. 5.
61 Prins, 'AIDS and global security', p. 940.

2 Severe acute respiratory syndrome

1 Y. Huang, *Mortal Peril: Public Health in China and its Security Implications*, Washington, DC: Chemical and Biological Arms Control Institute, 2003, p. 69.
2 J.S.M. Peiris, S.T. Lai, L.L.M. Poon, Y. Guan, L.Y.C. Yam, W. Lim, J. Nicholls, W.K.S. Yee, W.W. Yan and M.T. Cheung, 'Coronavirus as a possible cause of severe acute respiratory syndrome', *The Lancet* 361, 9366, 2003, 1319–1325.
3 S.V. Lawrence, 'The plague reaches much deeper', *Far Eastern Economic Review* 1 May 2003, 26–29, p. 26.
4 M. Curley and N. Thomas, 'Human security and public health in Southeast Asia: the SARS outbreak', *Australian Journal of International Affairs* 58, 1, 2004, 17–32, at p. 25.
5 *Joint Statement, ASEAN+3 Ministers of Health Special Meeting on SARS* (ASEAN

Online, 26 April 2003). Online, available at: www.aseansec.org/14745.htm (accessed 26 September 2005).

6 *Joint Declaration, Special ASEAN Leaders Meeting on Severe Acute Respiratory Syndrome (SARS)* (ASEAN Online, 29 April 2003). Online, available at: www.aseansec.org/14749.htm (accessed 26 September 2005).

7 *Joint Statement of the Special ASEAN-China Leaders Meeting on the Severe Acute Respiratory Syndrome (SARS)* (ASEAN Online, 29 April 2003). Online, available at: www.aseansec.org/14751.htm (accessed 26 September 2005).

8 Curley and Thomas, 'Human security and public health in Southeast Asia', pp. 27–28.

9 *Joint Statement of the Special ASEAN+3 Health Ministers Meeting on Severe Acute Respiratory Syndrome* (ASEAN Online, 11 June 2003). Online, available at: www.aseansec.org/14824.htm (accessed 26 September 2005).

10 M.-S. Ho and I.-J. Su, 'Preparing to prevent severe acute respiratory syndrome and other respiratory infections', *The Lancet Infectious Diseases* 4, 11, 2004, 684–689, p. 689.

11 Y.S. Wong and G. Chan, *The SAF SARS Diaries*, Singapore Armed Forces, 2004, pp. 27–28.

12 NIC, *SARS: Down But Still a Threat*, National Intelligence Council, 2003, p. 19.

13 Anonymous, *Malaysia Threatens Sick Passengers with Jail* (*Sydney Morning Herald* Online, 4 April 2003). Online, available at: www.smh.com.au/articles/2003/04/04/1048962932321.html (accessed 7 April 2003).

14 NIC, *SARS: Down But Still a Threat*, p. 12; WHO, *World Health Report 2003: Shaping the Future*, World Health Organization, 2003, p. 77.

15 Ho and Su, 'Preparing to prevent severe acute respiratory syndrome and other respiratory infections', p. 685.

16 J. deLisle, 'SARS, greater China, and the pathologies of globalisation and transition', *Orbis* 47, 4, 2003, 587–604, p. 598.

17 A. Freedman, 'SARS and regime legitimacy in China', *Asian Affairs* 36, 2, 2005, 169–180, p. 178.

18 J. deLisle, 'SARS, greater China, and the pathologies of globalisation and transition', p. 588, n582.

19 Editorial, 'Reflections on SARS', *The Lancet Infectious Diseases* 4, 11, 2004, 651.

20 M. Caballero-Anthony, 'SARS in Asia: crisis, vulnerabilities, and regional responses', *Asian Survey* 45, 3, 2005, 475–495, pp. 483–484.

21 E. Eckholm, 'SARS is the spark for a riot in China', *New York Times* 29 April 2003, A1; H.-F. Hung, 'The politics of SARS: containing the perils of globalization by more globalization', *Asian Perspective* 28, 1, 2004, 19–44, p. 41.

22 A.S. Ku and H.-L. Wang, 'The making and unmaking of civic solidarity: comparing the coping responses in Hong Kong and Taiwan during the SARS crisis', *Asian Perspective* 28, 1, 2004, 121–147, p. 136.

23 C. Cheng, 'To be paranoid is the standard? Panic responses to the SARS outbreak in the Hong Kong Special Administrative Region', *Asian Perspective* 28, 1, 2004, 67–98, p. 84.

24 Lawrence, 'The plague reaches much deeper', p. 27.

25 'Siracusa Principles on the limitation and derogation provisions in the international covenant on civil and political rights', *Human Rights Quarterly* 7, 1, 1985, 6.

26 D.P. Fidler, *SARS and International Law* (American Society of International Law Online, April 2003). Online, available at: www.asil.org/insights/insigh101.htm (accessed 10 October 2005).

27 Ho and Su, 'Preparing to prevent severe acute respiratory syndrome and other respiratory infections', p. 688.

28 Fidler, *SARS and International Law* (URL cited).
29 NIC, *SARS: Down But Still a Threat*, p. 20
30 N. Ma, 'SARS and the limits of the Hong Kong SAR administrative state', *Asian Perspective* 28, 1, 2004, 99–120, pp. 109, 113.
31 P.A. Tambyah, 'Severe acute respiratory syndrome from the trenches, at a Singapore university hospital', *The Lancet Infectious Diseases* 4, 11, 2004, 690–696, pp. 690, 692.
32 R. Borsuk and C. Prystay, 'Be prepared,' *Far Eastern Economic Review*, 21 August 2003, 34–35 at p. 35.
33 Anonymous, 'Our future with SARS,' *Far Eastern Economic Review*, 21 August 2003, 28–37 at p. 31.
34 Ku and Wang, 'The making and unmaking of civic solidarity', p. 131.
35 A.J. Bollet, *Plagues and Poxes: the Impact of Human History on Epidemic Disease*, New York: Demos, 2004, p. 227.
36 NIC, *SARS: Down But Still a Threat*, p. 22; WHO, *Summary of Probable SARS Cases with Onset of Illness from 1 November 2002 to 31 July 2003* (WHO Online, 26 September 2003). Online, available at: www.who.int/csr/sars/country/table2003_09_23/en/ (accessed 25 September 2005).
37 NIC, *SARS: Down But Still a Threat*, p. 22
38 Ku and Wang, 'The making and unmaking of civic solidarity', p. 135.
39 Curley and Thomas, 'Human security and public health in Southeast Asia', p. 29.
40 ABC, *Vietnam: SARS and a Lesson in Disease Control* (ABC News Online, 30 April 2003). Online, available at: www.abc.net.au/ra/asiapac/programs/s843022.htm (accessed 18 October 2005); Curley and Thomas, 'Human security and public health in Southeast Asia', p. 23.
41 Curley and Thomas, 'Human security and public health in Southeast Asia', pp. 24–25.

3 H5N1 avian influenza: pandemic pending?

1 A.J. McMichael, 'Human culture, ecological change, and infectious disease: are we experiencing history's fourth great transition?', *Ecosystem Health* 7, 2, 2001, 107–115, pp. 108–109.
2 WHO, *Ten Things You Need to Know about Pandemic Influenza* (WHO Online, 14 October 2005). Online, available at: www.who.int/csr/disease/influenza/pandemic10things/en/index.html (accessed 16 October 2005).
3 W. McKibbin and A. Sidorenko, *Global Macroeconomic Consequences of Pandemic Influenza*, Sydney: Lowy Institute for International Policy, 2006.
4 K. Stöhr and M. Esveld, 'Will vaccines be available for the next influenza pandemic?', *Science* 306, 5705, 2004, 2195–2196, p. 2195.
5 Anonymous, *Mysterious Disease Kills Thousands of Vietnamese Chickens* (*Sydney Morning Herald* Online, 7 January 2004). Online, available at: www.smh.com.au/articles/2004/01/06/1073268033540.html (accessed 12 January 2004).
6 OIE, *Update on Avian Influenza in Animals (Type H5)* (OIE Online, 4 September 2006). Online, available at: www.oie.int/downld/AVIAN%20INFLUENZA/A_AI-Asia.htm (accessed 19 September 2006).
7 WHO, *Confirmed Human Cases of Avian Influenza A (H5N1)* (WHO Online, 19 September 2006). Online, available at: www.who.int/csr/disease/avian_influenza/country/en/ (accessed 23 September 2006).
8 K. Ungchusak, P. Auewarakul, S.F. Dowell, R. Kitphati, W. Auwanit, P. Puthavathana, M. Uiprasertkul, K. Boonnak, C. Pittayawonganon, N.J. Cox, S.R. Zaki, P. Thawatsupha, M. Chittaganpitch, R. Khontong, J.M. Simmerman and

S. Chunsutthiwat, 'Probable person-to-person transmission of avian influenza A (H5N1)', *New England Journal of Medicine* 352, 4, 2005, 333–340.

9 A. Sipress, 'Bird flu in Indonesian family may raise global alert level', *Washington Post*, 25 May 2006, A21.

10 D.v. Riel, V.J. Munster, E.d. Wit, G.F. Rimmelzwaan, R.A.M. Fouchier, A.D.M.E. Osterhaus and T. Kuiken, 'H5N1 virus attachment to lower respiratory tract', *Science* 312, 2006, 399.

11 D. Lague, 'Stopping a killer', *Far Eastern Economic Review*, 5 February 2004, 12–16, pp. 15–16; A. Sipress, 'Indonesia neglected bird flu until too late, experts say', *Washington Post*, 20 October 2005, A01.

12 T. Palmer, *Indonesia Admits It Had Bird Flu Warning in November* (ABC News Online, 26 January 2004). Online, available at: www.abc.net.au/news/ newsitems/s1031950.htm (accessed 20 June 2004).

13 Anonymous, *Thailand Announces First Death from Bird Flu* (Sydney Morning Herald Online, 24 January 2004). Online, available at: www.smh.com.au/art- icles/2004/01/24/1074732634150.html (accessed 24 January 2004).

14 S.W. Crispin and T. McCawley, 'Did governments make it worse?', *Far Eastern Economic Review* 5 February 2004, 14–15, p. 14.

15 A. Sipress, 'Strategy on bird flu has human risks, officials say', *Washington Post*, 28 January 2004, A15.

16 Anonymous, *Bird Flu is Here to Stay, Say Experts* (Sydney Morning Herald Online, 9 August 2004). Online, available at: www.smh.com.au/articles/2004/08/08/ 1091903449874.html (accessed 16 October 2005).

17 D. MacKenzie, *Bird Flu Outbreak Started a Year Ago* (New Scientist Online, 28 January 2004). Online, available at: www.newscientist.com/article.ns?id=dn4614 (accessed 18 October 2005).

18 D. Normile, 'Vaccinating birds may help to curtail virus's spread', *Science* 306, 5695, 2004, 398–399, p. 399.

19 D. Mackenzie, *Vietnam in U-Turn over Bird Flu Vaccination* (New Scientist Online, 4 May 2005). Online, available at: www.newscientist.com/article.ns?id=dn7338 (accessed 10 October 2005).

20 J. Watts, 'Vietnam needs cash to stave off future outbreaks of bird flu', *The Lancet* 365, 9473, 2005, 1759–1760.

21 M. Cohen and B. McKay, 'Major flaws in flu detection', *Far Eastern Economic Review*, 12 February 2004, 18–20; D. Normile, 'Vietnam battles bird flu. and critics', *Science* 309, 5733, 2005, 368–373, p. 372.

22 K. Bradsher and L.K. Altman, 'Thais infected with bird flu; virus spreads', *New York Times*, 24 January 2004, A6.

23 BBC, *World Appeal to Contain Bird Flu* (BBC News Online, 27 January 2004). Online, available at: news.bbc.co.uk/1/hi/world/asia-pacific/3433509.stm (accessed 11 October 2005).

24 H. Chen, G. Deng, Z. Li, G. Tian, Y. Li, P. Jiao, L. Zhang, Z. Liu, R.G. Webster and K. Yu, 'The evolution of H5N1 influenza viruses in ducks in southern China', *Proceedings of the National Academy of Sciences* 101, 28, 2004, 10452–10457.

25 E. Nakashima, 'Officials urge farm overhauls to avert bird flu pandemic', *Washington Post*, 26 February 2005, A16; D. Normile, 'Ducks may magnify threat of avian flu virus', *Science* 306, 5698, 2004, 953.

26 R. Webster and D. Hulse, 'Controlling avian flu at the source', *Nature* 435, 7041, 2005, 415–416, p. 415.

27 D. Butler, '"Refusal to share" leaves agency struggling to monitor bird flu', *Nature* 435, 7039, 2005, 131.

28 M.H. Cheng, 'Cash boost for avian influenza exceeds expectations', *The Lancet* 367, 9507, 2006, 289.

29 Watts, 'Vietnam needs cash to stave off future outbreaks of bird flu', p. 1759.
30 WHO, *National Influenza Pandemic Plans* (WHO Online). Online, available at: www.who.int/csr/disease/influenza/nationalpandemic/en/index.html (accessed 2 September 2006).
31 A. Abbott, 'What's in the medicine cabinet?', *Nature* 435, 7041, 2005, 407–409, p. 409.
32 A. Sipress, 'Countries hit hard by bird flu have little medicine to treat humans', *Washington Post*, 6 July 2005, A09.
33 M. Enserink, 'Oseltamivir becomes plentiful – but still not cheap', *Science* 312, 2006, 382–383.
34 J. Kaiser, 'Facing down pandemic flu, the world's defenses are weak', *Science* 306, 5695, 2004, 394–397, p. 397.
35 A.S. Brett and A. Zuger, 'The run on Tamiflu – should physicians prescribe on demand?', *New England Journal of Medicine* 353, 25, 2005, 2636–2637.
36 M.D. de Jong, T.T. Thanh, T.H. Khanh, V.M. Hien, G.J.D. Smith, N.V. Chau, B.V. Cam, P.T. Qui, D.Q. Ha, Y. Guan, J.S.M. Peiris, T.T. Hien, and J. Farrar, 'Oseltamivir resistance during treatment of influenza A (H5N1) infection', *New England Journal of Medicine* 353, 25, 2005, 2667–2672.
37 I.M. Longini, Jr., A. Nizam, S. Xu, K. Ungchusak, W. Hanshaoworakul, D.A.T. Cummings and M.E. Halloran, 'Containing pandemic influenza at the source', *Science* 309, 5737, 2005, 1083–1087.
38 Australia, *Australian Health Management Plan for Pandemic Influenza*, Canberra: Commonwealth of Australia, 2006, p. 33.
39 Stöhr and Esveld, 'Will vaccines be available for the next influenza pandemic?', p. 2195.
40 M.T. Osterholm, 'A weapon the world needs', *Nature* 435, 7041, 2005, 417–418; B. Roberts and Y. Lu, 'Infectious diseases in Asia: implications for global health', in *AIDS in Asia*, Y. Lu and M. Essex (eds), New York: Kluwer, 2004, p. 395.
41 Kaiser, 'Facing down pandemic flu, the world's defenses are weak', p. 397.
42 Ibid., p. 394.
43 B.E. Zimmerman and D.J. Zimmerman, *Killer Germs: Microbes and Diseases That Threaten Humanity*, New York: Contemporary Books, 2003, p. 146.
44 WHO, *WHO Global Influenza Preparedness Plan*, Geneva: World Health Organization, 2005, p. 15.
45 Ibid. pp. 37, 41.
46 D. Cronin, 'Bird flu scary but not yet imminent', *Canberra Times* 22 October 2005, B4.
47 S. Levine, 'Leaders share flu pandemic concerns', *Washington Post* 7 November 2005, B01.
48 S. Tendler, *Flu Doctors to be Given Police Guards* (*The Times* Online, 2 November 2005). Online, available at: www.timesonline.co.uk/article/0,25149–|1853843,00.html (accessed 23 December 2005).
49 Australia, *Australian Health Management Plan for Pandemic Influenza*, p. 49.
50 W. Orent, 'The fear contagion', *Washington Post* 16 October 2005, B01.
51 D. Brown, 'Military's role in a flu pandemic', *Washington Post* 5 October 2005, A05.

4 Outbreak response: rallying around the state

1 N. Ma, 'SARS and the limits of the Hong Kong SAR administrative state', *Asian Perspective* 28, 1, 2004, 99–120, p. 112.
2 H. Cao, T. Nguyen and N. Daniels, 'HIV/AIDS and public health care in the greater Mekong River region', in *AIDS in Asia*, Y. Lu and M. Essex (eds), New York: Kluwer, 2004, pp. 62–63.

3 M.C. Lim-Quizon, 'HIV/AIDS in the Philippines', in *AIDS in Asia*, Y. Lu and M. Essex (eds), New York: Kluwer, 2004, p. 100.

4 H. Nomura and T. Nakayama, 'The Japanese healthcare system', *British Medical Journal* 331, 7518, 2005, 648–649.

5 V. Thamlikitkul, V. Tangcharoensathien and N. Bhamarapravati, 'Infectious diseases and the development of health systems in Thailand', in *AIDS in Asia*, Y. Lu and M. Essex (eds), New York: Kluwer, 2004, pp. 284, 287.

6 T. Kuiken, F.A. Leighton, R.A.M. Fouchier, J.W. LeDuc, J.S.M. Peiris, A. Schudel, K. Stohr and A.D.M.E. Osterhaus, 'Pathogen surveillance in animals', *Science* 309, 5741, 2005, 1680–1681.

7 J.-M. Kim, J. Lee and J.-S. Lee, 'The history of HIV and other infectious diseases in the Republic of Korea', in *AIDS in Asia*, Y. Lu and M. Essex (eds), New York: Kluwer, 2004, p. 310.

8 Cao, Nguyen and Daniels, 'HIV/AIDS and public health care in the greater Mekong River region', pp. 65–66.

9 K. Ahmad, 'Dengue death toll rises in Indonesia', *The Lancet* 363, 9413, 2004, 956; P. Das, 'Dengue in Indonesia', *The Lancet Infectious Diseases* 4, 4, 2004, 195.

10 A.S. Ku and H.-L. Wang, 'The making and unmaking of civic solidarity: comparing the coping responses in Hong Kong and Taiwan during the SARS crisis', *Asian Perspective* 28, 1, 2004, 121–147, p. 136.

11 K. Bradsher, *The Front Lines in the Battle Against Avian Flu are Running Short of Money* (*New York Times* Online, 9 October 2005). Online, available at: www.nytimes.com/2005/10/09/international/asia/09birdflu.html (accessed 9 October 2005).

12 J. Brower and P. Chalk, *The Global Threat of New and Reemerging Infectious Diseases: Reconciling US National Security and Public Health Policy*, Santa Monica: RAND, 2003, p. 104.

13 B. Guo, 'Transforming China's urban health-care system', *Asian Survey* 43, 2, 2003, 385–403, p. 399; D. Thompson, 'Pre-empting an HIV/AIDS disaster in China', *Seton Hall Journal of Diplomacy and International Relations* 4, 2, 2003, 29–44, pp. 30–31.

14 D. Blumenthal and W. Hsiao, 'Privatization and its discontents – the evolving Chinese health care system', *New England Journal of Medicine* 353, 11, 2005, 1165–1170, p. 1166.

15 Ibid., p. 1167.

16 Y. Huang, *Mortal Peril: Public Health in China and its Security Implications*, Washington, DC: Chemical and Biological Arms Control Institute, 2003, p. 15.

17 X. Xu, 'The impact of SARS on China', *Seton Hall Journal of Diplomacy and International Relations* 4, 2, 2003, 45–57, p. 52.

18 L. Wang, L. Kong, F. Wu, Y. Bai and R. Burton, 'Preventing chronic diseases in China', *The Lancet* 366, 9499, 2005, 1821–1824, p. 1822.

19 Huang, *Mortal Peril*, p. 15.

20 Ibid., pp. 70–71.

21 Editorial, 'China: towards "Xiaokang", but still living dangerously', *The Lancet* 363, 9407, 2004, 409.

22 Anonymous, 'A shot in the arm,' *Far Eastern Economic Review* 5 June 2003, 24–25, p. 24.

23 Blumenthal and Hsiao, 'Privatization and its discontents', p. 1169.

24 Japan, *Enhancing Capabilities for Responding to a Natural or Deliberate Epidemic of Infectious Diseases in Japan*, Meeting of Experts, Meeting of the States Parties to the Convention on the Prohibition of the Development, Production and Stockpiling of Bacteriological (Biological) and Toxin Weapons and on Their Destruction, 2004, p. 12.

25 ABC, *Australia Commits $100m to Bird Flu Fight* (ABC News Online, 19 November 2005). Online, available at: www.abc.net.au/news/newsitems/200511/s1510516.htm (accessed 30 December 2005).
26 *President Outlines Pandemic Influenza Preparations and Response* (White House Online, 1 November 2005). Online, available at: www.whitehouse.gov/news/releases/2005/11/print/20051101-1.html (accessed 9 November 2005).
27 Australia, *The Role of the World Health Organisation in Infectious Disease Surveillance: Australian Perspective*, Meeting of Experts, Meeting of the States Parties to the Convention on the Prohibition of the Development, Production and Stockpiling of Bacteriological (Biological) and Toxin Weapons and on Their Destruction, 2004, p. 4
28 *Fact Sheet on US–Singapore Regional Emerging Disease (REDI) Center* (US Department of Health and Human Services Online, 2004). Online, available at: www.globalhealth.gov/Singapore_REDI_MOU.shtml (accessed 25 May 2004).
29 J.W. Tappero, T. Siraprapasiri, W.C. Levine, S. Thanprasertsuk, S. Dowell, K. Limpakarnjanarat and T.D. Mastro, 'The Thailand MoPH–US CDC collaboration in Asia', in *AIDS in Asia*, Y. Lu and M. Essex (eds), New York: Kluwer, 2004, pp. 551, 553.
30 *Co-Chairs' Summary Report of the Meeting of the ASEAN Regional Forum Inter-Sessional Support Group on Confidence Building Measures* (ASEAN Online, 14 April 2004). Online, available at: www.aseansec.org/16096.htm (accessed 18 October 2005).
31 *Chairman's Statement of the 12th Meeting of the ASEAN Regional Forum* (ASEAN Regional Forum Online, 29 July 2005). Online, available at: www.aseanregional-forum.org/Default.aspx?tabid=67 (accessed 2 October 2005).
32 *APEC Emerging Infections Network* (University of Washington Online). Online, available at: depts.washington.edu/einet/ (accessed 31 October 2005).
33 *Busan Declaration, 13th APEC Economic Leaders' Meeting* (APEC Online, 18–19 November 2005). Online, available at: www.apec.org/apec/leaders__declarations/2005.html (accessed 29 December 2005).
34 WHO, *International Health Regulations* (WHO Online, 2006). Online, available at: www.who.int/csr/ihr/en/ (accessed 24 August 2006).
35 L.O. Gostin, 'International infectious disease law: revision of the World Health Organization's International Health Regulations', *Journal of the American Medical Association* 291, 21, 2004, 2623–2627, p. 2625.
36 D.P. Fidler, *Germs, Norms and Power: Global Health's Political Revolution* (Law, Social Justice & Global Development Online, 4 June 2004). Online, available at: www2.warwick.ac.uk/fac/soc/law/elj/lgd/2004_1/fidler/ (accessed 19 September 2006).
37 Kuiken *et al.*, 'Pathogen surveillance in animals', p. 1681.
38 WHO, *Public Health Response to Biological and Chemical Weapons: WHO Guidance* (WHO Online, 2004). Online, available at: www.who.int/csr/delibepidemics/biochemguide/en/ (accessed 13 February 2005).
39 US Senate Committee on Foreign Relations, 'The threat of bioterrorism and the spread of infectious diseases' (hearing transcript), 5 September 2001, p. 78.
40 *US Researchers Seeking Thai Help on Potentially Deadly Bacteria* (Global Security Newswire Online, 18 September 2003). Online, available at: www.nti.org/d_newswire/issues/newswires/2003_9_18.html#12 (accessed 19 September 2003).
41 *Final Document*, Fifth Review Conference of the States Parties to the Convention on the Prohibition of the Development, Production and Stockpiling of Bacteriological (Biological) and Toxin Weapons and on Their Destruction, 2002, pp. 3–4.
42 Australia, *Statement to the Biological Weapons Convention Meeting of States Parties,*

Meeting of the States Parties to the Convention on the Prohibition of the Development, Production and Stockpiling of Bacteriological (Biological) and Toxin Weapons and on Their Destruction, 2004.
43 Geneva, *Report of the Meeting of States Parties*, Meeting of the States Parties to the Convention on the Prohibition of the Development, Production and Stockpiling of Bacteriological (Biological) and Toxin Weapons and on Their Destruction, 2004, p. 4.
44 D. Normile, 'Who controls the samples?', *Science* 309, 5733, 2005, 372–373.

5 The science and history of deliberate disease

1 T.V. Inglesby, D.A. Henderson, J.G. Bartlett, M.S. Ascher, E. Eitzen, A.M. Friedlander, J. Hauer, J. McDade, M.T. Osterholm, T. O'Toole, G. Parker, T.M. Perl, P.K. Russell and K. Tonat, 'Anthrax as a biological weapon: medical and public health management', *Journal of the American Medical Association* 281, 18, 1999, 1735–1745, p. 1740.
2 E. Croddy, *Chemical and Biological Warfare: a Comprehensive Survey for the Concerned Citizen*, New York: Copernicus, 2002, pp. 206–207; M. Dando, 'Bioterrorism: what is the real threat?', Department of Peace Studies, University of Bradford, 2005, p. 14.
3 Dando, 'Bioterrorism', p. 12.
4 WHO, *Health Aspects of Chemical and Biological Weapons*, Geneva: World Health Organization, 1970, pp. 98–99.
5 OTA, *Proliferation of Weapons of Mass Destruction: Assessing the Risks*, Office of Technology Assessment, US Congress, 1993, pp. 53–55.
6 OTA, *Technologies Underlying Weapons of Mass Destruction*, Office of Technology Assessment, US Congress, 1993, pp. 93–94, 97.
7 Ibid. pp. 93–94.
8 Inglesby *et al.*, 'Anthrax as a biological weapon', p. 1744.
9 *Militarily Critical Technologies List (MCTL), Part 2: Weapons of Mass Destruction Technologies*, Office of the Under Secretary of Defense for Acquisition and Technology, 1998, p. II-3–7.
10 OTA, *Proliferation of Weapons of Mass Destruction*, p. 48.
11 C.W. Hedberg, J.B. Bender and D. Vesley, 'Protecting food, water, and ambient air', in *Terrorism and Public Health: a Balanced Approach to Strengthening Systems and Protecting People*, B.S. Levy and V.W. Sidel (eds), New York: Oxford University Press, 2003, pp. 310–312; R.M. Salerno, J. Gaudioso, R.L. Frerichs and D. Estes, 'A BW risk assessment: historical and technical perspectives', *Nonproliferation Review* 11, 3, 2004, 25–55, p. 44.
12 T.J. Torok, R.V. Tauxe, R.P. Wise, J.R. Livengood, R. Sokolow, S. Mauvais, K.A. Birkness, M.R. Skeels, J.M. Horan and L.R. Foster, 'A large community outbreak of salmonellosis caused by intentional contamination of restaurant salad bars', *Journal of the American Medical Association* 278, 5, 1997, 389–395.
13 Croddy, *Chemical and Biological Warfare*, p. 71.
14 'MCTL, Part 2', pp. II-1–1 to II-1–2.
15 R.R. Kiziah, 'Assessment of the emerging biocruise threat', in *The Gathering Biological Warfare Storm*, J.A. Davis and B.R. Schneider (eds), Westport: Praeger, 2004, p. 149.
16 'MCTL, Part 2', pp. II-1–2, II-1–35.
17 Cited in J.W. Powell, 'A hidden chapter in history', *Bulletin of the Atomic Scientists* 37, 8, 1981, 44–52, p. 51.
18 S.B. Martin, 'The role of biological weapons in international politics: the real military revolution', *Journal of Strategic Studies* 25, 1, 2002, 63–98, pp. 65–66.

19 M. Dando, *The New Biological Weapons: Threat, Proliferation and Control*, Boulder, CO: Lynne Rienner, 2001, p. 108.
20 Martin, 'The role of biological weapons in international politics', pp. 64, 80–81, 86.
21 An exception to the 'secret deterrent' paradox is Israel whose nuclear capability, although undeclared, appears to help deter large-scale attacks from neighbouring states.
22 G. Koblentz, 'Pathogens as weapons: the international security implications of biological warfare', *International Security* 28, 3, 2004, 84–122, p. 106.
23 Croddy, *Chemical and Biological Warfare*, p. 224; T. Mangold and J. Goldberg, *Plague Wars: a True Story of Biological Warfare*, London: Macmillan, 1999, pp. 17–18.
24 Mangold and Goldberg, *Plague Wars*, p. 16.
25 K. Alibek, *Biohazard*, London: Arrow, 1999, p. 166.
26 Croddy, *Chemical and Biological Warfare*, p. 225.
27 P. Williams and D. Wallace, *Unit 731: the Japanese Army's Secret of Secrets*, London: Hodder and Stoughton, 1989, pp. 26–27.
28 Ibid., p. 28.
29 Mangold and Goldberg, *Plague Wars*, p. 21.
30 Croddy, *Chemical and Biological Warfare*, p. 225.
31 Estimates of the number of Chinese deaths vary widely: see J. Ban, *Health, Security, and US Global Leadership*, Chemical and Biological Arms Control Institute, 2001, p. 18; D. Barenblatt, *A Plague Upon Humanity: the Hidden History of Japan's Biological Warfare Program*, New York: HarperCollins, 2004, p. xii; Z. Yunhua, 'China: balancing disarmament and development', in *Biological Warfare and Disarmament: New Problems/New Perspectives*, S. Wright (ed.), Lanham: Rowman and Littlefield, 2002, p. 214.
32 S. Endicott and E. Hagerman, *The United States and Biological Warfare: Secrets From the Early Cold War and Korea*, Bloomington, IN: Indiana University Press, 1998, pp. 37–38, 41.
33 Alibek, *Biohazard*, p. 37.
34 *US Paid Unit 731 Members for Data* (*Japan Times* Online, 15 August 2005). Online, available at: www.japantimes.co.jp/cgi-bin/makeprfy.pl5?nn20050815 a1.htm (accessed 16 August 2005).
35 J.W. Powell, 'A hidden chapter in history', *Bulletin of the Atomic Scientists* 37, 8, 1981, 44–52.
36 Williams and Wallace, *Unit 731*, p. 301.
37 Mangold and Goldberg, *Plague Wars*, p. 28.
38 Powell, 'A hidden chapter in history', p. 47.
39 Alibek, *Biohazard*, p. 233.
40 Cited in Powell, 'A hidden chapter in history', p. 48.
41 M. Leitenberg, 'Resolution of the Korean War biological warfare allegations', *Critical Reviews in Microbiology* 24, 3, 1998, 169–194, pp. 170, 172.
42 Endicott and Hagerman, *The United States and Biological Warfare*, p. x.
43 Ibid., p. 186.
44 H. Wilde and R.N. Johnson, 'Book review: *The United States and Biological Warfare: Secrets From the Early Cold War and Korea*', *Journal of the American Medical Association* 282, 19, 1999, 1877–1878.
45 Endicott and Hagerman, *The United States and Biological Warfare*, pp. 2–3.
46 See H. Wilde, 'Biological warfare in the 1940s and 1950s', *Journal of the American Medical Association* 284, 5, 2000, 562.
47 Endicott and Hagerman, *The United States and Biological Warfare*, pp. 188, 195.
48 Ibid., p. 195.

49 M. Leitenberg, 'New Russian evidence on the Korean War biological warfare allegations: background and analysis', *Cold War International History Project Bulletin* 11, 1998, 185–199, p. 187.
50 Ibid., p. 185.
51 K. Weathersby, 'Deceiving the deceivers: Moscow, Beijing, Pyongyang, and the allegations of bacteriological weapons use in Korea', *Cold War International History Project Bulletin*, 11, 1998, 176–185, pp. 176–177.
52 A. Selth, *Burma and Weapons of Mass Destruction, Working Paper 334*, Canberra: Strategic and Defence Studies Centre, Australian National University, 1999.
53 Ibid., p. 3.
54 Ibid., pp. 10–12.
55 E.D. Harris, 'Threat reduction and North Korea's CBW programs', *Nonproliferation Review* 11, 3, 2004, 86–109, p. 189.
56 CIA, *Unclassified Report to Congress on the Acquisition of Technology Relating to Weapons of Mass Destruction and Advanced Conventional Munitions, 1 July Through 31 December 2003* (CIA Online, November 2004). Online, available at: www.cia.gov/cia/reports/721_reports/july_dec2003.htm (accessed 30 December 2005).
57 Harris, 'Threat reduction and North Korea's CBW programs', p. 89.
58 *North Korea Profile: Biological Facilities* (Nuclear Threat Initiative Online, April 2003). Online, available at: www.nti.org/e_research/profiles/NK/Biological/print/57_276.prt (accessed 22 July 2005).
59 Harris, 'Threat reduction and North Korea's CBW programs', pp. 89–90.
60 K.-S. Kim, 'North Korea's CB weapons: threat and capability', *Korean Journal of Defense Analysis* 14, 1, 2002, 69–95, p. 84.
61 Croddy, *Chemical and Biological Warfare*, p. 53.
62 Spore-forming agents like *B. anthracis* can better withstand the shock of artillery delivery: 'MCTL, Part 2', p. II-1–59.
63 J.S. Bermudez, *Shield of the Great Leader: the Armed Forces of North Korea*, Sydney: Allen and Unwin, 2001, p. 150.
64 *Proliferation: Threat and Response*, Office of the Secretary of Defense, 2001, p. 13.
65 Kiziah, 'Assessment of the emerging biocruise threat', p. 162.
66 WHO, *Country Health Profile – DPR Korea* (WHO Southeast Asia Regional Office Online, 29 October 2003). Online, available at: w3.whosea.org/cntry-health/dprkorea/index.htm (accessed 22 July 2005).
67 *Proliferation: Threat and Response*, p. 15
68 J. Miller, S. Engelberg and W. Broad, 'US germ warfare research pushes treaty limits', *New York Times*, 4 September 2001, A1.
69 CIA, *Unclassified Report to Congress on the Acquisition of Technology Relating to Weapons of Mass Destruction and Advanced Conventional Munitions* (URL cited).
70 *Proliferation: Threat and Response*, p. 17
71 'MCTL, Part 2', p. II-1–36.
72 A. Mauroni, *Chemical and Biological Warfare: a Reference Handbook*, Santa Barbara: ABC-CLIO, 2003, p. 64; MIIS, *Chemical and Biological Weapons: Possession and Programs Past and Present* (Monterey Institute of International Studies Online, 9 April 2002). Online, available at: cns.miis.edu/research/cbw/possess.htm (accessed 1 September 2006), *Taiwan Overview* (Nuclear Threat Initiative Online, January 2003). Online, available at: www.nti.org/e_research/e1_taiwan_1.html#biological (accessed 1 November 2003).
73 CBS, *Secret Weapon vs. Taiwan's SARS* (CBS News Online, 20 May 2003). Online, available at: www.cbsnews.com/stories/2003/05/20/health/main554764.shtml (accessed 13 May 2005); W. Minnick, 'Taiwan's secret research unveiled', *Jane's Defence Weekly*, 4 June 2003, 13.
74 Mauroni, *Chemical and Biological Warfare*, p. 65.

6 Biological attacks and the non-state perpetrator

1 This chapter is a revised version of: Christian Enemark, 'Biological attacks and the non-state actor: a threat assessment', *Intelligence and National Security* 21, 6, 2006. Permission to republish kindly granted by Taylor and Francis (www.tandf.co.uk/journals/titles/02684527.asp).

2 J. Stern, 'Dreaded risks and the control of biological weapons', *International Security* 27, 3, 2002, 89–123, pp. 104, 121.

3 M.B.A. Oldstone, *Viruses, Plagues, and History*, New York: Oxford University Press, 1998, pp. 29–30.

4 A.J. Bollet, *Plagues and Poxes: the Impact of Human History on Epidemic Disease*, New York: Demos, 2004, p. 206; J. Stern, 'The prospect of domestic bioterrorism', *Emerging Infectious Diseases* 5, 4, 1999, 517–522, pp. 518–519.

5 See A. Dolnik and J. Pate, 'Mass casualty terrorism: understanding the bioterrorist threat', in *The Changing Face of Terrorism*, R. Gunaratna (ed.), Singapore: Eastern Universities Press, 2004, p. 109; G. Koblentz, 'Pathogens as weapons: the international security implications of biological warfare', *International Security* 28, 3, 2004, 84–122, p. 103, A.M. Muir, 'Terrorism and weapons of mass destruction: the case of Aum Shinrikyo', *Studies in Conflict and Terrorism* 22, 1, 1999, 79–97, p. 81; Stern, 'The prospect of domestic bioterrorism', p. 521; J.B. Tucker, 'Historical trends related to bioterrorism: an empirical analysis', *Emerging Infectious Diseases* 5, 4, 1999, 498–504, p. 503.

6 T.J. Torok, R.V. Tauxe, R.P. Wise, J.R. Livengood, R. Sokolow, S. Mauvais, K.A. Birkness, M.R. Skeels, J.M. Horan and L.R. Foster, 'A large community outbreak of salmonellosis caused by intentional contamination of restaurant salad bars', *Journal of the American Medical Association* 278, 5, 1997, 389–395, p. 390.

7 D.S. Gressang, 'Audience and message: assessing terrorist WMD potential', *Terrorism and Political Violence* 13, 3, 2001, 83–106, pp. 185, 190.

8 Ibid., pp. 98–100.

9 J. Parachini, 'Putting WMD terrorism into perspective', *Washington Quarterly* 26, 4, 2003, 37–50, p. 45.

10 M.T. Osterholm and J. Schwarz, *Living Terrors: What America Needs to Know to Survive the Coming Bioterrorist Catastrophe*, New York: Delacourt Press, 2000, pp. 24, 78, 91.

11 *Dark Winter Overview* (University of Pittsburgh Medical Center Online, 2001). Online, available at: www.upmc-biosecurity.org/pages/events/dark_winter/dark_winter.html (accessed 31 December 2005).

12 *Atlantic Storm Scenario Assumptions* (Atlantic Storm Online, 14 January 2005). Online, available at: www.atlantic-storm.org/materials/assumptions.html (accessed 31 December 2005).

13 ABC, *Biowar* (ABC Online, 4 September 2005). Online, available at: www.abc.net.au/rn/talks/bbing/stories/s1450124.htm (accessed 8 September 2005).

14 W. Laqueur, *The New Terrorism: Fanaticism and the Arms of Mass Destruction*, New York: Oxford University Press, 1999, p. 65.

15 M. Dando, *Bioterrorism: What is the Real Threat?*, Department of Peace Studies, University of Bradford, 2005, p. 27.

16 R. Danzig, *Catastrophic Bioterrorism – What is to be Done?* Washington, DC: National Defense University, 2003, p. 2.

17 A. Haselkorn, 'Iraq's biowarfare option: last resort, pre-emption, or a blackmail weapon?', *Biosecurity and Bioterrorism* 1, 1, 2003, 19–26, p. 24.

18 See, for example, Dolnik and Pate, 'Mass casualty terrorism', p. 112; J. Gearson, 'The nature of modern terrorism', in *Superterrorism: Policy Responses*, L. Freedman (ed.), Oxford: Blackwell, 2002, p. 21; Muir, 'Terrorism and weapons of mass

destruction', p. 86, Stern, 'The prospect of domestic bioterrorism', p. 522, J.B. Tucker, 'Biological threat assessment: is the cure worse than the disease?', *Arms Control Today* 34, 2004, 13–19, pp. 13–14.

19 G. Matsumoto, 'Anthrax powder: state of the art?', *Science* 302, 5650, 2003, 1492–1497, p. 1493.

20 M. Leitenberg, 'Biological weapons and bioterrorism in the first years of the twenty-first century', *Politics and the Life Sciences* 21, 2, 2002, 3–27, p. 19.

21 J. Miller, S. Engelberg and W. Broad, *Germs: the Ultimate Weapon*, Sydney: Simon & Schuster, 2001, pp. 297–298.

22 CIA, *Terrorist CBRN: Material and Effects*, Central Intelligence Agency, 2003, p. 2.

23 G. Alcorn, *Crop Spraying: Techniques and Equipment*, Sydney: Inkata Press, 1993, pp. 85–87; E. Croddy, *Chemical and Biological Warfare: a Comprehensive Survey for the Concerned Citizen*, New York: Copernicus, 2002, p. 82.

24 D.B. Levin and G.V.d. Amorim, 'Potential for aerosol dissemination of biological weapons: lessons from biological control of insects', *Biosecurity and Bioterrorism* 1, 1, 2003, 37–42, p. 41.

25 T.V. Inglesby, D.A. Henderson, J.G. Bartlett, M.S. Ascher, E. Eitzen, A.M. Friedlander, J. Hauer, J. McDade, M.T. Osterholm, T. O'Toole, G. Parker, T.M. Perl, P.K. Russell and K. Tonat, 'Anthrax as a biological weapon: medical and public health management', *Journal of the American Medical Association* 281, 18, 1999, 1735–1745, p. 1737.

26 M. Enserink, 'How devastating would a smallpox attack really be?', *Science* 296, 5573, 2002, 1592–1595, p. 1592.

27 M.L. Wheelis, 'Investigations of suspicious outbreaks of disease', in *Biological Warfare: Modern Offense and Defense*, R.A. Zilinskas (ed.), Boulder, CO: Lynne Rienner, 2000, p. 109.

28 Dolnik, 'Die and let die: exploring links between suicide terrorism and terrorist use of chemical, biological, radiological, and nuclear weapons', *Studies in Conflict and Terrorism* 26, 1, 2003, 17–35, p. 20.

29 Ibid., p. 30.

30 *Bio-Terror Text Seized in JI Raid* (*The Australian* Online, 21 October 2003). Online, available at: www.theaustralian.news.com.au/printpage/0,5942,7616369, 00.html (accessed 21 October 2003); *Traces of 'Bio-weapons' Found in Philippines* (Straits Times Online, 20 October 2003). Online, available at: straitstimes.asia1.com.sg/storyprintfriendly/0,1887,215594,00.html (accessed 21 October 2003).

31 *Philippines Says No Bio-Chem Traces at JI Hideout* (Reuters Online, 22 October 2003). Online, available at: www.alertnet.org/thenews/newsdesk/MAN102821. htm (accessed 23 October 2003).

32 *Literature on Chemical Arms Seized from Abu Sayyaf Man* (*Manila Times* Online, 23 May 2004). Online, available at: www.manilatimes.net/national/2004/may/23/ yehey/metro/20040523met1.html (accessed 27 May 2004).

33 Abdel-Aziz, *The Mujahideen Poisons Handbook* (The Disease.Net Online, 1996). Online, available at: www.thedisease.net/arcana/nbc/chemical/Mujahideen_ Poisons.pdf (accessed 21 August 2005).

34 CIA, *Unclassified Report to Congress on the Acquisition of Technology Relating to Weapons of Mass Destruction and Advanced Conventional Munitions, 1 July Through 31 December 2003* (CIA Online, November 2004). Online, available at: www.cia.gov/ cia/reports/721_reports/july_dec2003.htm (accessed 30 December 2005).

35 CBS, *Is Al Qaeda Making Anthrax?* (CBS News Online, 9 October 2003). Online, available at: www.cbsnews.com/stories/2003/10/09/eveningnews/ main577395.shtml (accessed 27 June 2004).

36 C.A. Thayer, 'Political terrorism in Southeast Asia', *Pointer* 29, 4, 2003, 53–62, pp. 56–60.
37 Muir, 'Terrorism and weapons of mass destruction', p. 83; W. Rosenau, 'Aum Shinrikyo's biological weapons program: why did it fail?', *Studies in Conflict and Terrorism* 24, 4, 2001, 289–301, p. 291.
38 K.B. Olson, 'Aum Shinrikyo: once and future threat?', *Emerging Infectious Diseases* 5, 4, 1999, 513–516, p. 515.
39 Leitenberg, 'Biological weapons and bioterrorism', p. 12; Miller, Engelberg and Broad, *Germs*, p. 160; Olson, 'Aum Shinrikyo', p. 515; Parachini, 'Putting WMD terrorism into perspective', p. 42.
40 Rosenau, 'Aum Shinrikyo's biological weapons program', p. 289, A.P. Schmid, 'Terrorism and the use of weapons of mass destruction: from where the risk?', in *The Future of Terrorism*, M. Taylor and J. Horgan (eds), London: Frank Cass, 2000, pp. 124–125.
41 Rosenau, 'Aum Shinrikyo's biological weapons program', p. 293.
42 K. Alibek, *Biohazard*, London: Arrow, 1999, p. 278.
43 H. Takahashi, P. Keim, A.F. Kaufmann, C. Keys, K.L. Smith, K. Taniguchi, S. Inouye and T. Kurata, 'Bacillus anthracis incident, Kameido, Tokyo, 1993', *Emerging Infectious Diseases* 10, 1, 2004, 117–120.
44 Rosenau, 'Aum Shinrikyo's biological weapons program', p. 291.
45 T. Ballard, J. Pate, G. Ackerman, D. McCauley and S. Lawson, *Chronology of Aum Shinrikyo's CBW Activities* (Monterey Institute of International Studies Online, 15 March 2001). Online, available at: cns.miis.edu/pubs/reports/aum_chrn.htm (accessed 16 August 2005).
46 Muir, 'Terrorism and weapons of mass destruction', p. 88; Rosenau, 'Aum Shinrikyo's biological weapons program', p. 296.
47 Miller, Engelberg and Broad, *Germs*, p. 154.

7 Responses to the biological weapons problem

1 *South Korean Response: New Defense Unit Begins Operations* (Global Security Newswire Online, 1 February 2002). Online, available at: www.nti.org/d_newswire/issues/2002/2/1/10s.html (accessed 21 November 2003).
2 Japan, *Enhancing Capabilities for Responding to a Natural or Deliberate Epidemic of Infectious Diseases in Japan*, Meeting of Experts, Meeting of the States Parties to the Convention on the Prohibition of the Development, Production and Stockpiling of Bacteriological (Biological) and Toxin Weapons and on Their Destruction, 2004, p. 6; P. Kallender, 'Rising to meet terror threat', *Defense News* 5 May 2003, 18.
3 NAS, *Chemical and Biological Terrorism: Research and Development to Improve Civilian Medical Response*, Washington, DC: National Academy of Sciences, 1999, p. 13.
4 *Tokyo Holds Anti-Biological Attack Drill* (Yahoo News Online, 1 December 2003). Online, available at: uk.news.yahoo.com/031201/325/efb3u.html (accessed 1 September 2005).
5 T.J. Torok, R.V. Tauxe, R.P. Wise, J.R. Livengood, R. Sokolow, S. Mauvais, K.A. Birkness, M.R. Skeels, J.M. Horan and L.R. Foster, 'A large community outbreak of salmonellosis caused by intentional contamination of restaurant salad bars', *Journal of the American Medical Association* 278, 5, 1997, 389–395, p. 393.
6 *National Strategy to Combat Weapons of Mass Destruction* (White House Online, December 2002). Online, available at: www.whitehouse.gov/news/releases/2002/12/WMDStrategy.pdf (accessed 28 August 2005).
7 D.G. Gompert, 'Sharpen the fear', *Bulletin of the Atomic Scientists* 56, 1, 2000, 22–23, pp. 22–23.

8 R.R. Kiziah, 'Assessment of the emerging biocruise threat', in *The Gathering Biological Warfare Storm*, J.A. Davis and B.R. Schneider (ed.), Westport, CT: Praeger, 2004, p. 130.

9 *Proliferation Security Initiative (PSI): Interdiction Principles* (Australian Department of Foreign Affairs and Trade Online). Online, available at: www.dfat.gov.au/globalissues/psi/ (accessed 6 October 2003).

10 S. Haeri, *WMD Transport Targeted on High Seas* (Asia Times Online, 12 September 2003). Online, available at: www.atimes.com/atimes/Korea/EI12Dg01.html (accessed 24 November 2003).

11 S. Sakamaki and D. Struck, 'Japan cracks down on firms tied to N. Korea', *Washington Post* 22 May 2003, A23.

12 CIA, *Unclassified Report to Congress on the Acquisition of Technology Relating to Weapons of Mass Destruction and Advanced Conventional Munitions, 1 July Through 31 December 2003* (CIA Online, November 2004). Online, available at: www.cia.gov/cia/reports/721_reports/july_dec2003.htm (accessed 30 December 2005).

13 Chapter One, *Report to the President of the United States* (Commission on the Intelligence Capabilities of the United States Regarding Weapons of Mass Destruction Online, 31 March 2005). Online, available at: www.wmd.gov/report/wmd_report.pdf (accessed 21 May 2005).

14 Ibid.

15 CIA and DIA, *Iraqi Mobile Biological Warfare Agent Production Plants*, Central Intelligence Agency and Defense Intelligence Agency, 2003, pp. 1–4.

16 J. Miller and W.J. Broad, 'Some analysts of Iraq trailers reject germ use', *New York Times* 7 June 2003, A1.

17 CIA and DIA, *Iraqi Mobile Biological Warfare Agent Production Plants*, p. 5.

18 D. Jehl, 'Iraqi trailers said to make hydrogen, not biological arms', *New York Times* 9 August 2003, A1.

19 CIA and DIA, *Iraqi Mobile Biological Warfare Agent Production Plants*, p. 1.

20 C. Deulfer, *Trailers Suspected of Being Mobile BW Agent Production Units, Comprehensive Report of the Special Advisor to the DCI on Iraq's WMD* (CIA Online, 30 September 2004). Online, available at: www.cia.gov/cia/reports/iraq_wmd_2004/chap6_annxD.html (accessed 3 September 2005).

21 M. Dando, 'Genomics, bioregulators, cell receptors and potential biological weapons', *Defense Analysis* 17, 3, 2001, 239–258, p. 242; *Technologies Underlying Weapons of Mass Destruction*, Office of Technology Assessment, US Congress, 1993, p. 116.

22 J.-w. Guo and X.-s. Yang, 'Ultramicro, nonlethal, and reversible: looking ahead to military biotechnology', *Military Review* July–August 2005, 75–78.

23 *Final Document*, Fifth Review Conference of the States Parties to the Convention on the Prohibition of the Development, Production and Stockpiling of Bacteriological (Biological) and Toxin Weapons and on Their Destruction, 2002, pp. 3–4.

24 P. Moore, *Killer Germs: Rogue Diseases of the Twenty-First Century*, London: Carlton, 2001, p. 1.

25 VERTIC, *Time to Lay Down the Law: the Status of National Laws to Enforce the BWC*, Verification Research, Training and Information Centre, 2003, p. 11.

26 D. Ruppe, *BWC: Survey Finds Many Nations Lacking Required Treaty Legislation* (Global Security Newswire Online, 13 August 2003). Online, available at: www.nti.org/d_newswire/issues/thisweek/2003_8_14_biow.html (accessed 17 August 2003).

27 *1540 Committee, List of Submitting Member States* (UN Online, 1 August 2006). Online, available at: disarmament2.un.org/Committee1540/report.html (accessed 3 September 2006).

28 VERTIC, *Time to Lay Down the Law*, p. 42.
29 R.o. Korea, *Note Verbale Dated 27 October 2004 from the Permanent Mission of the Republic of Korea to the United Nations Addressed to the Chairman of the Committee* (1540 Committee, UN Online, 27 October 2004). Online, available at: www.un.org/Docs/journal/asp/ws.asp?m=S/AC.44/2004/(02)/24 (accessed 31 December 2005).
30 China, *A Compiled List of Laws and Regulations of China in Relation to the Implementation of the Biological Weapons Convention*, Meeting of the States Parties to the Convention on the Prohibition of the Development, Production and Stockpiling of Bacteriological (Biological) and Toxin Weapons and on Their Destruction, 2003.
31 China, *Letter Dated 2 September 2005 from the Permanent Representative of China to the United Nations Addressed to the Chairman of the Committee* (1540 Committee, UN Online, 2 September 2005). Online, available at: www.un.org/Docs/journal/asp/ws.asp?m=S/AC.44/2004/(02)/4/Add.1 (accessed 31 December 2005).
32 Japan, *National Paper*, Meeting of the States Parties to the Convention on the Prohibition of the Development, Production and Stockpiling of Bacteriological (Biological) and Toxin Weapons and on Their Destruction, 2003, pp. 2–3.
33 Japan, *Note Verbale dated 17 March 2006 from the Permanent Mission of Japan to the United Nations Addressed to the Chairman of the Committee* (1540 Committee, UN Online, 17 March 2006). Online, available at: www.un.org/Docs/journal/asp/ws.asp?m=S/AC.44/2004/(02)/49/Add.1 (accessed 31 August 2006).
34 Brunei, *Note Verbale Dated 30 December 2004 from the Permanent Mission of Brunei Darussalam to the United Nations Addressed to the Chairman of the Committee* (1540 Committee, UN Online, 30 December 2004). Online, available at: www.un.org/Docs/journal/asp/ws.asp?m=S/AC.44/2004/(02)/96 (accessed 31 December 2005).
35 *Malaysia, Legislative Action to Implement the Obligations under the Convention on the Prohibition of the Development, Production and Stockpiling of Bacteriological (Biological) and Toxin Weapons and on Their Destruction*, Meeting of the States Parties to the Convention on the Prohibition of the Development, Production and Stockpiling of Bacteriological (Biological) and Toxin Weapons and on Their Destruction, 2003.
36 Malaysia, *Note Verbale Dated 26 October 2004 from the Permanent Mission of Malaysia to the United Nations Addressed to the Chairman of the Committee* (1540 Committee, UN Online, 26 October 2004). Online, available at: www.un.org/Docs/journal/asp/ws.asp?m=S/AC.44/2004/(02)/35 (accessed 31 December 2005).
37 VERTIC, *Biological Weapons Convention: Collection of National Implementation Legislation* (VERTIC Online, 2003). Online, available at: www.vertic.org/datasets/bwlegislation.html (accessed 3 September 2005).
38 Laos, *Note Verbale Dated 3 May 2005 from the Permanent Mission of the Lao People's Democratic Republic to the United Nations Addressed to the Chairman of the Committee* (1540 Committee, UN Online, 3 May 2005). Online, available at: www.un.org/Docs/journal/asp/ws.asp?m=S/AC.44/2004/(02)/117 (accessed 31 December 2005).
39 Indonesia, *Letter Dated 22 November 2005 from the Deputy Permanent Representative of the Permanent Mission of Indonesia to the United Nations Addressed to the Chairman of the Committee* (1540 Committee, UN Online, 22 November 2005). Online, available at: www.un.org/Docs/journal/asp/ws.asp?m=S/AC.44/2004/(02)/45/Add.1 (accessed 31 December 2005).
40 *Draft Biological Agents and Toxins Bill* (Singapore Ministry of Health Online,

11 April 2005). Online, available at: www.moh.gov.sg/cmaweb/attachments/ press/361b4c0568N5/Draft_BATA.pdf (accessed 30 May 2005).

41 Vietnam, *Note Verbale Dated 26 October 2004 from the Permanent Mission of Vietnam to the United Nations Addressed to the Chairman of the Committee* (1540 Committee, UN Online, 26 October 2004). Online, available at: www.un.org/Docs/journal/ asp/ws.asp?m=S/AC.44/2004/(02)/39 (accessed 31 December 2005).

42 Thailand, *Note Verbale Dated 5 November 2004 from the Permanent Mission of Thailand to the United Nations Addressed to the Chairman of the Committee* (1540 Committee, UN Online, 5 November 2004). Online, available at: www.un.org/ Docs/journal/asp/ws.asp?m=S/AC.44/2004/(02)/71 (accessed 31 December 2005).

43 *Guidelines for Transfers of Sensitive Chemical or Biological Items* (Australia Group Online, June 2004). Online, available at: www.australiagroup.net/en/ guidelines.html (accessed 31 December 2005).

44 P.R. Chari and G. Deshingkar, 'Putting teeth in the BWC: an Indian view', *Politics and the Life Sciences* 18, 1, 1999, 86–91, p. 88.

45 *2005 Australia Group Plenary* (Australia Group Online, April 2005). Online, available at: www.australiagroup.net/en/releases/press_2005.htm (accessed 21 August 2005).

46 *Statement by Mr Toshio Sano, Representative of the Delegation of Japan*, Fifth Review Conference of the States Parties to the Convention on the Prohibition of the Development, Production and Stockpiling of Bacteriological (Biological) and Toxin Weapons and on Their Destruction, 2001.

47 *Statement by Ambassador Chung Eui-yong, Permanent Representative of the Republic of Korea*, Fifth Review Conference of the States Parties to the Convention on the Prohibition of the Development, Production and Stockpiling of Bacteriological (Biological) and Toxin Weapons and on Their Destruction, 2001.

48 *Statement of Ambassador Sha Zukang, Head of the Chinese Delegation*, Fifth Review Conference of the States Parties to the Convention on the Prohibition of the Development, Production and Stockpiling of Bacteriological (Biological) and Toxin Weapons and on Their Destruction, 2001.

49 Z. Yunhua, 'China: balancing disarmament and development', in *Biological Warfare and Disarmament: New Problems/New Perspectives*, S. Wright (ed.), Lanham: Rowman and Littlefield, 2002, pp. 224, 231.

50 China, *Foreign Ministry Spokesman Liu Jianchao's Remarks on China's Renewed Control List of Regulations on Export Control of Dual-Use Biological Agents and Related Equipment and Technologies* (Chinese Ministry of Foreign Affairs Online, 1 August 2006). Online, available at: www.fmprc.gov.cn/eng/xwfw/s2510/2535/ t265668.htm (accessed 31 August 2006); *Regulations of the People's Republic of China on Export Control of Dual Use Biological Agents and Related Equipment and Technologies* (Nuclear Threat Initiative Online, 14 October 2002). Online, available at: www.nti.org/db/china/engdocs/bioregs_1002.htm (accessed 13 December 2003).

51 China, *Letter Dated 4 October 2004 from the Permanent Representative of China to the United Nations Addressed to the Chairman of the Committee* (1540 Committee, UN Online, 4 October 2004). Online, available at: www.un.org/Docs/journal/asp/ ws.asp?m=S/AC.44/2004/(02)/4 (accessed 31 December 2005).

52 N. Wisnumurti, *Statement by Head of Delegation of the Republic of Indonesia*, Fifth Review Conference of the States Parties to the Convention on the Prohibition of the Development, Production and Stockpiling of Bacteriological (Biological) and Toxin Weapons and on Their Destruction, 2001.

53 Y. Huang, *Mortal Peril: Public Health in China and its Security Implications*, Washington, DC: Chemical and Biological Arms Control Institute, 2003, p. 2.

54 E.J. Lord, 'Exercises involving an act of biological or chemical terrorism: what are the psychological consequences?', *Military Medicine* 166, Supplement 2, 2001, 34–35.
55 A.E. Norwood, 'Psychological effects of biological warfare', *Military Medicine* 166, Supplement 2, 2001, 27–28; V. Ramalingaswarmi, 'Psychosocial effects of the 1994 plague outbreak in Surat, India', *Military Medicine* 166, Supplement 2, 2001, 29–30.
56 WHO, *Preparedness for the Deliberate Use of Biological Agents: a Rational Approach to the Unthinkable*, Geneva: World Health Organization, 2002, pp. 2–4.
57 UN, *A More Secure World: Our Shared Responsibility. Report of the High-Level Panel on Threats, Challenges and Change*, United Nations, 2004, p. 47.
58 R. Brookmeyer, E. Johnson and R. Bollinger, 'Public health vaccination policies for containing an anthrax outbreak', *Nature* 432, 7019, 2004, 901–904.

8 Beyond biosafety: the security consciousness of scientists

1 *The Biotechnology Promise: Capacity-Building for Participation of Developing Countries in the Bioeconomy*, United Nations, 2004, pp. 38, 40; L.T. Hickok and R.M. Salerno, *Time to Wake up to Bioterror Threat* (*Straits Times* Online, 26 January 2004). Online, available at: straitstimes.asia1.com.sg/storyprintfriendly/0,1887,231848,00.html (accessed 29 January 2004).
2 G.W. Christopher, T.J. Cieslak, J.A. Pavin and E.M. Eitzen, 'Biological warfare: a historical perspective', *Journal of the American Medical Association* 278, 5, 1997, 412–417, p. 416.
3 A. Goldstein, 'Scientist is watched for sign of Ebola', *Washington Post* 20 February 2004, B02; J. Miller, 'Russian scientist dies in Ebola accident at former weapons lab', *New York Times* 25 May 2004, A9.
4 See, for example, F. James, 'Anti-bioterror labs raise risk to US, critics say', *Chicago Tribune* 5 December 2004, 9; J. Kaiser, 'Citizens sue to block Montana biodefense lab', *Science* 305, 5687, 2004, 1088.
5 D. Normile and G. Vogel, 'Early indications point to lab infection in new SARS case', *Science* 301, 5640, 2003, 1642–1643.
6 WHO, *Biosafety and SARS incident in Singapore, September 2003*, WHO Western Pacific Regional Office, 2003, pp. 12–14.
7 Ibid., p. 6.
8 D. Normile, 'Second lab accident fuels fears about SARS', *Science* 303, 2004, 26; *Taiwan's New SARS Case Raises Questions about Sloppy Procedures* (USA Today Online, 17 December 2003). Online, available at: www.usatoday.com/news/health/2003-12-17-singapore-sars_x.htm# (accessed 9 May 2005).
9 BBC, *China Finds Suspected SARS Case* (BBC News Online, 22 April 2004). Online, available at: news.bbc.co.uk/2/hi/asia-pacific/3649897.stm (accessed 31 December 2005); D. Murphy, 'Lab bungle', *Far Eastern Economic Review* 6 May 2004, 18; J. Yardley and L.K. Altman, 'China is scrambling to curb SARS cases after a death', *New York Times* 24 April 2004, 4.
10 J. Yardley, 'China expands quarantine in aggressive effort to contain SARS', *New York Times* 27 April 2004, 5.
11 W. Chung-ming, *Taiwan Government Mobilizes against Contagious Disease* (Taiwan News Online, 24 April 2004). Online, available at: www.etaiwannews.com/Taiwan/2004/04/24/1082776673.htm (accessed 25 April 2004).
12 M. Enserink and L. Du, 'SARS: China dumps CDC head, probes lab', *Science* 305, 5681, 2004, 163; WHO, *Chinese Ministry of Health Summary of China's Investigation into the April Outbreak* (WHO Western Pacific Regional Office Online, 2 July 2004). Online, available at: www.wpro.who.int/sars/docs/update/update_07022004_revisedfinal.asp (accessed 1 May 2005).

13 Malaysia, *Legislative Action to Implement the Obligations under the Convention on the Prohibition of the Development, Production and Stockpiling of Bacteriological (Biological) and Toxin Weapons and on Their Destruction*, Meeting of the States Parties to the Convention on the Prohibition of the Development, Production and Stockpiling of Bacteriological (Biological) and Toxin Weapons and on Their Destruction, 2003, p. 2.

14 Indonesia, *Note Verbale Dated 28 October 2004 from the Permanent Mission of Indonesia to the United Nations Addressed to the Chairman of the Committee* (1540 Committee, UN Online, 28 October 2004). Online, available at: www.un.org/Docs/journal/asp/ws.asp?m=S/AC.44/2004/(02)/45 (accessed 31 December 2005).

15 Japan, *National Paper Prepared by Japan*, Meeting of the States Parties to the Convention on the Prohibition of the Development, Production and Stockpiling of Bacteriological (Biological) and Toxin Weapons and on Their Destruction, 2003, p. 5.

16 Ibid., pp. 4–5.

17 China, *A Compiled List of Laws and Regulations of China in Relation to the Implementation of the Biological Weapons Convention*, Meeting of the States Parties to the Convention on the Prohibition of the Development, Production and Stockpiling of Bacteriological (Biological) and Toxin Weapons and on Their Destruction, 2003, pp. 2, 4.

18 M. Guihua, 'China revises law on infectious diseases', *The Lancet Infectious Diseases* 4, 11, 2004, 652.

19 China, *National Implementation Measures and Biosecurity and Oversight Mechanisms: Practice and Proposals*, Meeting of the States Parties to the Convention on the Prohibition of the Development, Production and Stockpiling of Bacteriological (Biological) and Toxin Weapons and on Their Destruction, 2003, p. 3.

20 *Anthrax, Resistant TB Not Stored Properly at Many Japanese Labs* (Japan Today Online, 7 October 2005). Online, available at: www.japantoday.com/e/?content=news&id=351256 (accessed 7 October 2005).

21 Cao, 'SARS: "Waterloo" of Chinese science', *China: an International Journal* 2, 2, 2004, 262–286, p. 283.

22 *Draft Biological Agents and Toxins Bill* (Singapore Ministry of Health Online, 11 April 2005). Online, available at: www.moh.gov.sg/cmaweb/attachments/press/361b4c0568N5/Draft_BATA.pdf (accessed 30 May 2005).

23 *A Survey of Asian Life Scientists: the State of Biosciences, Laboratory Biosecurity, and Biosafety in Asia* (Sandia National Laboratories Online, February 2006). Online, available at: www.biosecuritycodes.org/docs/Asia%20summary%20SAND%20report%20final.pdf (accessed 23 August 2006).

24 *Annual CBM Declarations* (Biological and Toxin Weapons Convention Online). Online, available at: www.opbw.org/cbms/annual_cbm.htm (accessed 4 September 2006).

25 *Anthrax III: Chronology of Outbreak and Investigation* (Global Security Newswire Online, 21 December 2001). Online, available at: www.nti.org/d_newswire/issues/newswires/2001_12_21.html#10 (accessed 27 June 2003).

26 T.D. Read, S.L. Salzberg, M. Pop, M. Shumway, L. Umayam, L. Jiang, E. Holtzapple, J.D. Busch, K.L. Smith, J.M. Schupp, D. Solomon, P. Keim and C.M. Fraser, 'Comparative genome sequencing for discovery of novel polymorphisms in Bacillus anthracis', *Science* 296, 5575, 2002, 2028–2033.

27 G. Gugliotta, 'Still no arrests in anthrax probe, but "progress" is noted', *Washington Post* 4 August 2002, A08.

28 E. Choffnes, 'Bioweapons: new labs, more terror?', *Bulletin of the Atomic Scientists* 58, 5, 2002, 29–32, p. 29; J. Guillemin, *Biological Weapons: From the Invention of State-Sponsored Programs to Contemporary Bioterrorism*, New York: Columbia

University Press, 2005, p. 175; G. Matsumoto, 'Anthrax powder: state of the art?', *Science* 302, 5650, 2003, 1492–1497; J.B. Tucker, 'Biological threat assessment: is the cure worse than the disease?', *Arms Control Today* 34, 2004, 13–19, p. 15.

29 G. Gugliotta, 'Still no arrests in anthrax probe, but "progress" is noted', A08.

30 J. Miller, 'Scientist files suit over anthrax inquiry', *New York Times* 27 August 2003, A13.

31 A. Lengel, 'Little progress in FBI probe of anthrax attacks', *Washington Post* 16 September 2005, A01.

32 B. Kellman, 'Biological terrorism: legal measures for preventing catastrophe', *Harvard Journal of Law and Public Policy* 24, 2, 2001, 417–488, p. 450.

33 *List of Select Biological Agents and Toxins* (CDC Online, 5 May 2005). Online, available at: www.cdc.gov/od/sap/docs/salist.pdf (accessed 5 July 2005).

34 J. Gaudioso and R.M. Salerno, 'Biosecurity and research: minimizing adverse impacts', *Science* 304, 5671, 2004, 687.

35 United States Code, Title 18, Chapter 10 (Biological Weapons), section 175b(b)(2).

36 K. Chang, '30 plague vials put career on the line', *New York Times* 19 October 2003, p. 32; Gaudioso and Salerno, 'Biosecurity and research', p. 687; K. Hoyt and S.G. Brooks, 'A double-edged sword: globalization and biosecurity', *International Security* 28, 3, 2004, 123–148, p. 141.

37 B.E. Murray, K.E. Anderson, K. Arnold, J.G. Bartlett, C.C. Carpenter, S. Falkow, J.T. Hartman, T. Lehman, T.W. Reid, F.M. Ryburn, Jr., R.B. Sack, M.J. Struelens, L.S. Young and W.B. Greenough III, 'Destroying the life and career of a valued physician-scientist who tried to protect us from plague: was it really necessary?', *Clinical Infectious Diseases* 40, 11, 2005, 1644–1648.

38 M. Enserink and D. Malakoff, 'The trials of Thomas Butler', *Science* 302, 5653, 2003, 2054–2063, p. 2057.

39 Chang, '30 plague vials put career on the line', p. 32.

40 Enserink and Malakoff, 'The trials of Thomas Butler', pp. 2057–2058.

41 Chang, '30 plague vials put career on the line', p. 32, Murray *et al.*, 'Destroying the life and career of a valued physician-scientist', p. 1645.

42 Chang, '30 plague vials put career on the line', p. 32, M. Larkin, 'Arrest spurs alert about "Select Agents" regulations', *The Lancet Infectious Diseases* 3, 3, 2003, 120.

43 Murray *et al.*, 'Destroying the life and career of a valued physician-scientist', p. 1645.

44 *University Professor Faces Broad Set of Charges Stemming From Plague Incident* (Global Security Newswire Online, 4 September 2003). Online, available at: www.nti.org/d_newswire/issues/newswires/2003_9_4.html#12 (accessed 5 September 2003).

45 C. Connolly, 'Science groups protest researcher's treatment', *Washington Post* 28 August 2003, A02.

46 C. Piller, 'Plague expert cleared of serious charges in bioterror case', *Los Angeles Times* 2 December 2003, A16.

47 Editorial, 'Mr Butler and the Law', *Washington Post* 25 September 2003, A32.

48 K. Chang, 'Scientist in plague case is sentenced to two years', *New York Times* 11 March 2004, 18; Piller, 'Plague expert cleared of serious charges in bioterror case', A16.

49 *United States v Butler*, 5:03-C.R.-037-C (US District Court, Northern District of Texas Online, 10 March 2004). Online, available at: www.fas.org/butler/sentence.html (accessed 19 May 2005).

50 *Letter in Defense of Butler from the Presidents of the National Academy of Sciences and*

Institute of Medicine to Attorney General John Ashcroft (Federation of American Scientists Online, 15 August 2003). Online, available at: www.fas.org/sgp/news/2003/08/nas081503.pdf (accessed 19 May 2005).

51 Murray *et al.*, 'Destroying the life and career of a valued physician-scientist', p. 1646.

52 Enserink and Malakoff, 'The trials of Thomas Butler', p. 2054; Murray *et al.*, 'Destroying the life and career of a valued physician-scientist', p. 1647.

53 *Letter in Defense of Butler* (URL cited).

54 See, for example, R.M. Atlas and J. Reppy, 'Globalizing biosecurity', *Biosecurity and Bioterrorism* 3, 1, 2005, 51–60; M. Barletta, A. Sands and J.B. Tucker, 'Keeping track of anthrax: the case for a Biosecurity Convention', *Bulletin of the Atomic Scientists* 58, 3, 2002, 57–62; J.D. Steinbruner and E.D. Harris, 'Controlling dangerous pathogens', *Issues in Science and Technology* 19, 3, 2003, 47–54, p. 53.

55 Atlas and Reppy, 'Globalizing biosecurity', pp. 51, 55; J.B. Tucker, *Biosecurity: Limiting Terrorist Access to Deadly Pathogens*, Washington, DC: United States Institute of Peace, 2003, p. 37.

56 *Final Document*, Fourth Review Conference of the States Parties to the Convention on the Prohibition of the Development, Production and Stockpiling of Bacteriological (Biological) and Toxin Weapons and on Their Destruction, 1996, p. 17.

57 *Final Document*, Fifth Review Conference of the States Parties to the Convention on the Prohibition of the Development, Production and Stockpiling of Bacteriological (Biological) and Toxin Weapons and on Their Destruction, 2002, pp. 3–4.

58 *Report of the Meeting of States Parties, Volume 1*, Meeting of the States Parties to the Convention on the Prohibition of the Development, Production and Stockpiling of Bacteriological (Biological) and Toxin Weapons and on Their Destruction, 2003, p. 5.

59 Malaysia, *Legislative Action to Implement the Obligations under the Convention on the Prohibition of the Development, Production and Stockpiling of Bacteriological (Biological) and Toxin Weapons and on Their Destruction*, p. 3.

60 China, *A Compiled List of Laws and Regulations of China in Relation to the Implementation of the Biological Weapons Convention*, p. 1.

61 Japan, *National Paper Prepared by Japan*, pp. 3–4.

62 Japan, *Possible Measures for Strengthening Biosecurity*, Meeting of the States Parties to the Convention on the Prohibition of the Development, Production and Stockpiling of Bacteriological (Biological) and Toxin Weapons and on Their Destruction, 2003, p. 2.

63 S. Wright and S. Ketcham, 'The problem of interpreting the US biological defense research program', in *Preventing a Biological Arms Race*, S. Wright (ed.), Cambridge, MA: MIT Press, 1990, pp. 171–172.

64 See H.C. Kelly, 'Terrorism and the biology lab', *New York Times* 2 July 2003, A25; M. Moodie, *Reducing the Biological Threat: New Thinking, New Approaches*, Washington, DC: Chemical and Biological Arms Control Institute, 2003, p. 41.

65 N. Munro, *Scientific Community Struggles to Balance Openness, Security* (Global Security Newswire Online, 5 September 2003). Online, available at: www.nti.org/d_newswire/issues/newswires/2003_9_5.html#10 (accessed 9 September 2003).

66 NAS, *Biotechnology Research in an Age of Terrorism*, National Academy of Sciences, 2004, p. 5.

67 R.J. Jackson, A.J. Ramsay, C.D. Christensen, S. Beaton, D.F. Hall and I.A. Ramshaw, 'Expression of mouse Interleukin-4 by a recombinant ectromelia virus

suppresses cytolytic lymphocyte responses and overcomes genetic resistance to mousepox', *Journal of Virology* 75, 3, 2001, 1205–1210.

68 J. Cello, A.V. Paul and E. Wimmer, 'Chemical synthesis of poliovirus cDNA: generation of infectious virus in the absence of natural template', *Science* 297, 5583, 2002, 1016–1018.

69 Australia, *Codes of Conduct for Scientists: Considerations during a BWC Regional Workshop and Subsequent Reflections*, Meeting of Experts, Meeting of the States Parties to the Convention on the Prohibition of the Development, Production and Stockpiling of Bacteriological (Biological) and Toxin Weapons and on Their Destruction, 2005, p. 3.

70 G.L. Epstein, 'Controlling biological warfare threats: resolving potential tensions among the research community, industry, and the national security community', *Critical Reviews in Microbiology* 27, 4, 2001, 321–354, p. 343.

71 NAS, *Biotechnology Research in an Age of Terrorism*, pp. 4–9.

72 J. Couzin, 'US agencies unveil plan for biosecurity peer review', *Science* 303, 5664, 2004, 1595; *HHS Will Lead Government-Wide Effort to Enhance Biosecurity in 'Dual Use' Research* (US Department of Health and Human Services Online, 4 March 2004). Online, available at: www.hhs.gov/news/press/2004pres/20040304.html (accessed 27 May 2005).

73 R. Casagrande, 'Biological warfare targeted at livestock', *BioScience* 52, 7, 2002, 577–581.

74 'Statement on the consideration of biodefence and biosecurity', *Nature* 421, 6925, 2003, 771.

75 T.M. Tumpey, C.F. Basler, P.V. Aguilar, H. Zeng, A. Solorzano, D.E. Swayne, N.J. Cox, J.M. Katz, J.K. Taubenberger, P. Palese and A. Garcia-Sastre, 'Characterization of the reconstructed 1918 Spanish influenza pandemic virus', *Science* 310, 5745, 2005, 77–80.

76 J. Kaiser, 'Resurrected influenza virus yields secrets of deadly 1918 pandemic', *Science* 310, 5745, 2005, 28–29.

77 P.A. Sharp, '1918 flu and responsible science', *Science* 310, 5745, 2005, 17.

78 J. Cohen, 'HHS asks PNAS to pull bioterrorism paper', *Science* 308, 5727, 2005, 1395.

79 L.M. Wein, 'Got toxic milk?', *New York Times* 30 May 2005, A15.

80 L.M. Wein and Y. Liu, 'Analyzing a bioterror attack on the food supply: the case of botulinum toxin in milk', *Proceedings of the National Academy of Sciences* 102, 28, 2005, 9984–9989.

81 B. Alberts, 'Modelling attacks on the food supply', *Proceedings of the National Academy of Sciences* 102, 28, 2005, 9737–9738, p. 9737.

82 A. McCook, *PNAS Publishes Bioterror Paper, After All* (*The Scientist* Online, 29 June 2005). Online, available at: www.the-scientist.com/news/20050629/01 (accessed 1 July 2005).

83 S. Shane, 'Paper describes potential poisoning of milk', *New York Times* 29 June 2005, A20.

84 Munro, *Scientific Community Struggles to Balance Openness, Security* (URL cited).

85 W. Broad, D. Johnston and J. Miller, 'Subject of anthrax inquiry tied to anti-germ training', *New York Times* 2 July 2003, A1; M.W. Thompson, 'Hatfill trained US team on bioweapons', *Washington Post* 3 July 2003, A03.

86 *Draft Recommendations for a Code of Conduct for Biodefense Programs* (Federation of American Scientists Online, November 2002). Online, available at: www.fas.org/bwc/papers/code.pdf (accessed 30 May 2005).

9 Biodefence: lessons from the United States

1 Sections of this chapter were originally published as: Christian Enemark, 'United States biodefense, international law, and the problem of intent', *Politics and the Life Sciences* 24, 1–2, 2005, 32–42. Permission to republish kindly granted by the editor-in-chief of that journal.

2 C. Lam, C. Franco and A. Schuler, 'Billions for biodefense: federal agency biodefense funding, FY2006-FY2007', *Biosecurity and Bioterrorism* 4, 2, 2006, 113–127, p. 114.

3 J. Guillemin, *Biological Weapons: From the Invention of State-Sponsored Programs to Contemporary Bioterrorism*, New York: Columbia University Press, 2005, p. 199.

4 J. Fiorill, *US Plans to Defend Against Engineered Bioattack* (Global Security Newswire Online, 15 June 2005). Online, available at: www.nti.org/d_newswire/issues/2005/6/15/F1EB5240–6C65–41F5-A24E-DFD8EFF6C642.html (accessed 1 July 2005).

5 *Biotechnology, Weapons and Humanity II*, London: British Medical Association, 2004, 69.

6 T. Clarke and J. Knight, 'Fast vaccine offers hope in battle with Ebola', *Nature* 424, 6949, 2003, 602; N.J. Sullivan, T.W. Geisbert, J.B. Geisbert, L. Xu, Z.-y. Yang, M. Roederer, R.A. Koup, P.B. Jahrling and G.J. Nabel, 'Accelerated vaccination for Ebola virus haemorrhagic fever in non-human primates', *Nature* 424, 6949, 2003, 681–684.

7 T.W. Geisbert, L.E. Hensley, P.B. Jahrling, T. Larsen, J.B. Geisbert, J. Paragas, H.A. Young, T.M. Fredeking, W.E. Rote and G.P. Vlasuk, 'Treatment of Ebola virus infection with a recombinant inhibitor of factor VIIA/tissue factor: a study in rhesus monkeys', *The Lancet* 362, 9400, 2003, 1953–1958.

8 *NIAID Awards First $27 Million Using New Bioshield Authorities* (NIH Online, 9 May 2005). Online, available at: www.nih.gov/news/pr/may2005/niaid-09.htm (accessed 9 June 2005).

9 *NIAID Funds Construction of Biosafety Laboratories* (NIAID Online, 30 September 2003). Online, available at: www2.niaid.nih.gov/newsroom/releases/nblscorrect21.htm (accessed 10 May 2005).

10 M. Enserink and J. Kaiser, 'Has biodefense gone overboard?', *Science* 307, 5714, 2005, 1396–1398, p. 1396.

11 'An open letter to Elias Zerhouni', *Science* 307, 5714, 2005, 1409–1410.

12 Editorial, 'An Acidic Message', *Washington Post* 10 March 2005, A20.

13 See R. Loeppky, ' "Biomania" and US foreign policy', *Millennium* 34, 1, 2005, 85–113.

14 S. Wright and S. Ketcham, 'The problem of interpreting the US biological defense research program', in *Preventing a Biological Arms Race*, S. Wright (ed.), Cambridge, MA: MIT Press, 1990, pp. 176–177.

15 Guillemin, *Biological Weapons*, p. 200.

16 M. Leitenberg, 'Distinguishing offensive from defensive biological weapons research', *Critical Reviews in Microbiology* 29, 3, 2003, 223–257, p. 248.

17 Cited in Guillemin, *Biological Weapons*, pp. 202–203.

18 S. Shane, *Bioterror Fight May Spawn New Risks* (Baltimore Sun Online, 27 June 2004). Online, available at: www.baltimoresun.com/news/nationworld/bal-te.biodefense27jun27,0,6098679.story (accessed 29 June 2004).

19 R. Nelson, 'Biosafety laboratories proliferate across the USA', *The Lancet Infectious Diseases* 4, 10, 2004, 596.

20 Shane, *Bioterror Fight May Spawn New Risks* (URL cited).

21 N. Schwellenbach, 'Biodefense: a plague of researchers', *Bulletin of the Atomic Scientists* 61, 3, 2005, 14–16.

22 NAS, *Biotechnology Research in an Age of Terrorism*, National Academy of Sciences, 2004, p. 3.
23 B. Knickerbocker, *Concern over Spread of Biodefense Labs* (*Christian Science* Monitor Online, 25 September 2003). Online, available at: www.csmonitor.com/2003/0925/p02s01–uspo.html (accessed 14 July 2004).
24 Shane, *Bioterror Fight May Spawn New Risks* (URL cited).
25 J.B. Tucker, *Scourge: the Once and Future Threat of Smallpox*, New York: Atlantic Monthly Press, 2001, p. 145.
26 A.E. Cha, 'Computers simulate terrorism's extremes', *Washington Post* 4 July 2005, A01.
27 H.A. Kissinger, *National Security Decision Memorandum (NSDM) 35, United States Policy on Chemical Warfare Program and Bacteriological/Biological Research Program, from National Security Advisory Henry A. Kissinger to the Vice President, the Secretary of State, the Secretary of Defense, etc., November 25, 1969* (George Washington University National Security Archive Online, 7 December 2001). Online, available at: www.gwu.edu/~nsarchiv/NSAEBB/NSAEBB58/RNCBW8.pdf (accessed 27 May 2005).
28 Anonymous, 'The Scowcroft Memorandum', *CBW Conventions Bulletin*, 57, 2002, 2.
29 Leitenberg, 'Distinguishing offensive from defensive biological weapons research', p. 242.
30 *Fact Sheet: National Biodefense Analysis and Countermeasures Center* (US Department of Homeland Security Online, 24 February 2005). Online, available at: www.dhs.gov/dhspublic/display?content=4336 (accessed 13 April 2005).
31 J. Warrick, 'The secretive fight against bioterror', *Washington Post* 30 July 2006, A01.
32 G. Korch, *Leading Edge of Biodefense: the National Biodefense Analysis and Countermeasures Center, Lecture to the Department of Defense Pest Management Workshop, Jacksonville Naval Air Station, 9 February 2004* (Bioweapons and Biodefense Freedom of Information Fund Online, 2004). Online, available at: www.cbw-transparency.org/archive/nbacc.pdf (accessed 26 May 2005).
33 *Militarily Critical Technologies List (MCTL), Part 2: Weapons of Mass Destruction Technologies*, Office of the Under Secretary of Defense for Acquisition and Technology, 1998, p. II-3–7.
34 *Adherence to and Compliance with Arms Control, Nonproliferation, and Disarmament Agreements and Commitments* (US Department of State Online, 30 August 2005). Online, available at: www.state.gov/t/vci/rls/rpt/51977.htm#chapter6 (accessed 22 December 2005).
35 CBDP, *Chemical and Biological Defense Program Annual Report to Congress*, US Department of Defense, 2006, p. 69.
36 Ibid. p. 70.
37 J. Miller, S. Engelberg and W. Broad, 'US germ warfare research pushes treaty limits', *New York Times* 4 September 2001, A1.
38 J. Miller, S. Engelberg and W. Broad, *Germs: the Ultimate Weapon*, Sydney: Simon & Schuster, 2001.
39 Ibid., p. 295.
40 Ibid., p. 288.
41 D. Ruppe, *Proposed US Biological Research Could Challenge Treaty Restrictions, Experts Charge* (Global Security Newswire Online, 30 June 2004). Online, available at: www.nti.org/d_newswire/issues/2004_6_30.html#8736549A (accessed 21 April 2005).
42 *Draft Recommendations for a Code of Conduct for Biodefense Programs* (Federation of American Scientists Online, November 2002). Online, available at: www.fas.org/bwc/papers/code.pdf (accessed 30 May 2005).

43 Miller, Engelberg and Broad, *Germs*, p. 298.
44 Anonymous, 'US approves development of enhanced anthrax', *Arms Control Today* 31, 9, 2001, 26; A.P. Pomerantsev, N.A. Staritsin, Y.V. Mockov and L.I. Marinin, 'Expression of cereolysine AB genes in Bacillus anthracis vaccine strain ensures protection against experimental hemolytic anthrax infection', *Vaccine* 15, 17/18, 1997, 1846–1850.
45 Miller, Engelberg and Broad, *Germs*, p. 309.
46 CBDP, *Chemical and Biological Defense Program Annual Report to Congress*, US Department of Defense, 2005, pp. 49–50.
47 Ibid., p. 61.
48 Ibid., p. 62.
49 Wright and Ketcham, 'The problem of interpreting the US biological defense research program', p. 177.
50 R.J. Jackson, A.J. Ramsay, C.D. Christensen, S. Beaton, D.F. Hall and I.A. Ramshaw, 'Expression of mouse Interleukin-4 by a recombinant ectromelia virus suppresses cytolytic lymphocyte responses and overcomes genetic resistance to mousepox', *Journal of Virology* 75, 3, 2001, 1205–1210.
51 R. Roos, *Scientists Research Antidotes to Super Mousepox Virus* (University of Minnesota Online, 6 November 2003). Online, available at: www.cidrap.umn.edu/cidrap/content/bt/smallpox/news/nov0603mousepox.html (accessed 8 November 2003).
52 S. Wright, *Taking Biodefense Too Far* (*Bulletin of the Atomic Scientists* Online, November/December 2004). Online, available at: www.thebulletin.org/issues/2004/nd04/nd04wright.html (accessed 1 November 2004).
53 D. Smith, 'Call to stop deadly viruses getting into wrong hands', *Sydney Morning Herald*, 29 December 2003, 5; *US Develops Lethal New Viruses* (*New Scientist* Online, 29 October 2003). Online, available at: www.newscientist.com/article.ns?id=dn4318 (accessed 5 November 2003).
54 Wright, *Taking Biodefense Too Far* (URL cited).
55 CBDP, 'CBDP 2005 Report to Congress', p. 61.
56 Wright, *Taking Biodefense Too Far* (URL cited).
57 J.B. Tucker, 'Biological threat assessment: is the cure worse than the disease?', *Arms Control Today* 34, 2004, 13–19, p. 18.
58 *Annex to Final Declaration on Confidence Building Measures*, Third Review Conference of the States Parties to the Convention on the Prohibition of the Development, Production and Stockpiling of Bacteriological (Biological) and Toxin Weapons and on Their Destruction, 1991.
59 *Biotechnology, Weapons and Humanity II*, British Medical Association, 2004, p. 112.
60 K. Alibek, *Biohazard*, London: Arrow, 1999, p. 234.
61 *Draft Recommendations for a Code of Conduct for Biodefense Programs* (URL cited).
62 *United States, Annual CBM Return* (Biological and Toxin Weapons Convention Online, April 2004). Online, available at: www.opbw.org/cbms/annual_cbms/USA_cbm_2004.pdf (accessed 5 September 2006).
63 W. Broad, 'Book says pre-Gulf War discovery raised germ warfare fears', *New York Times* 7 June 1998, A6.
64 M. Kelley and J. Coghlan, 'Mixing bugs and bombs', *Bulletin of the Atomic Scientists* 59, 5, 2003, 24–31.
65 Tucker, 'Biological threat assessment', p. 14.
66 V. Futrakul, *Statement of the Permanent Representative of Thailand*, Fifth Review Conference of the States Parties to the Convention on the Prohibition of the Development, Production and Stockpiling of Bacteriological (Biological) and Toxin Weapons and on Their Destruction, 2001.
67 *HHS, Republic of Korea Expand Cooperation on Infectious Diseases Research* (US

Department of Health and Human Services Online, 22 July 2003). Online, available at: www.hhs.gov/news/press/2003pres/20030722a.html (accessed 24 July 2003).

68 *Fact Sheet on US–Singapore Regional Emerging Disease (REDI) Center* (US Department of Health and Human Services Online, 2004). Online, available at: www.globalhealth.gov/Singapore_REDI_MOU.shtml (accessed 25 May 2004).

69 China, *China's Non-Proliferation Policy and Measures* (Chinese Ministry of Foreign Affairs Online, 3 December 2003). Online, available at: www.fmprc.gov.cn/eng/zxxx/t54978.htm (accessed 13 December 2003).

70 *Statement of Ambassador Sha Zukang, Head of the Chinese Delegation*, Fifth Review Conference of the States Parties to the Convention on the Prohibition of the Development, Production and Stockpiling of Bacteriological (Biological) and Toxin Weapons and on Their Destruction, 2001.

Index

Milton Keynes UK
Ingram Content Group UK Ltd.
UKHW040103071024
449327UK00019B/768

9 780415 569897